D0508801

REGNANCY
AND FITNESS

CHERRY BAKER

all you need to
know to exercise
safely and effectively
throughout pregnancy

PREGNANCY
AND FITNESS

A & C Black • London

First published 2006 by
A & C Black Publishers Ltd
38 Soho Square, London W1D 3HB
www.acblack.com

Copyright © 2006 Cherry Baker

ISBN-10: 0 7136 6916 0
ISBN-13: 978 0 7136 6919 9

A CIP catalogue record for this book is available from the British Library.

Note: Whilst every effort has been made to ensure that the content of this book is technically accurate and as sound as possible, neither the author nor the publishers can accept responsibility for any injury or loss sustained as a result of use of this material.

Acknowledgements
Cover photograph © Getty Images
Photographs on pages 1, 47, 85, 90, 91, 97, 99, 117, 147 © Corbis. Food images (pages 149–160) © Comstock Images.
All other photographs © Grant Pitchard
Illustrations by James Wakelin
Inside Design by Jo Grey

A & C Black uses paper produced with elemental chlorine-free pulp, harvested from managed sustainable forests.

Printed and bound in China by C & C Offset Printing Co., Ltd.

contents

Acknowledgements

Many people have taught me along the way about exercise and pregnancy. Too many to mention here but those of you who have crossed my path over the years with all your knowledge will know who you are – thank you!

To my three girls Esther, Freya and Enya for giving me real hands on experience about exercising throughout pregnancy. My proudest creations!

Thank you to all the teaching team at The Studio for all the cover you did and to Emma H (my right hand).

To my fantastic, gorgeous John who slept without me so many nights while I was up writing the book.

To my brilliant family and friends who never see me or hear from me when working on projects such as this but are still there at the end and support me throughout.

To all the models in the book and to all the pregnant mums who have worked with me.

And last but not least to all at A&C Black.

The models

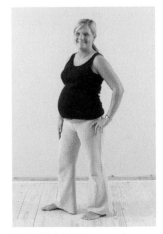

Kath Walsh at 29 weeks with her second baby

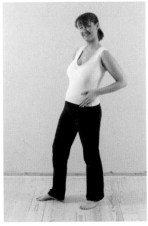

Samantha Wise at 23 weeks with her second baby

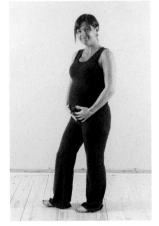

Nicky Whitehurst at 28 weeks with her second baby

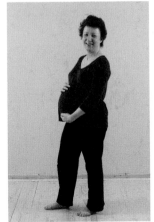

Maeve Moorcroft at 38 weeks with her first baby

Preface

You may have many reasons for reading this book. Perhaps you are planning to be pregnant or are already pregnant. You may have a relative, partner or friend that is pregnant. Perhaps you are an exercise or health professional working with mums-to-be. Whatever the reason you have for reading this book, I hope it is useful.

My main hope in writing this book is that it helps in some way to make your experience of pregnancy a positive one. I wish you all the luck in the world with this most miraculous and wonderful experience. I am constantly amazed by the human body – it is quite possibly the best piece of machinery ever! The female human form and the physical adaptations it makes naturally through pregnancy are nothing less than brilliant, and they constantly fill me with awe and inspiration. This has inspired me over the years to learn all I can about exercise and pregnancy and to share this with the students I teach and, of course, the mums-to-be that attend my classes.

Cherry Baker
October 2005

Introduction

Many pregnant women want to continue to exercise throughout their pregnancy to maintain their fitness levels, prepare for the birth and allow themselves a quick recovery. But as your body will be changing rapidly every day, your usual approach to exercise will also need to adapt to support your changing body and developing baby.

Exercising through your pregnancy has many positive benefits, and as long as the exercise is appropriate for each stage of pregnancy, it should not be detrimental to the health and well-being of you or your growing baby. Unfortunately many pregnant women are still given conflicting information about pregnancy and exercise, causing confusion about exactly what type of exercise can and can't be done. *Pregnancy and Fitness* works towards answering all your questions and more. By giving you the facts about the anatomical and physiological changes you are experiencing and how these relate to exercise it aims to eliminate the guesswork and worry about the rights and wrongs of exercising during pregnancy.

Pregnancy is time of great change, both physical and psychological. It is a specific condition that needs extra care and consideration when participating in exercise, and you will need to make changes to your exercise programme throughout your pregnancy. However, many of you may be amazed to discover how much exercise you can actually do when pregnant. You may also find that your friends, relatives and partner may be against you exercising, or think that you are going to harm your unborn baby. If this is the case, sit them down over a long weekend and ask them to read this book. If it helps to keep them focused, supply the odd glass of wine and promise a treat of some kind if they actually finish the book!

Every mum-to-be wants the best for their unborn baby, and this book will also help you to understand that exercise is only part of the picture in trying to stay healthy and fit during your pregnancy. Eating correctly and resting sufficiently are also essential aspects of a healthy and positive pregnancy.

I once had the pleasure to work with a lovely Irish midwife called Mary, who uttered one of the most practical statements about pregnancy that I have ever come across; it was simple and yet sound advice:

> *'If you were running a marathon in nine months time, you would train for the event. However, the physical training is only part of the picture. You would also have to eat well, stay well hydrated and get enough rest to enable you to prepare for the event ahead.*
>
> *Pregnancy is no different to this. You need to exercise correctly, eat well and take sufficient rest to allow yourself to prepare for the birth.'*

However, it is also important to say that no matter how much you plan and prepare throughout your pregnancy, the labour and birth of your child will very rarely be an easy event. Every woman will have a a very individual and unique experience throughout their pregnancy and labour. Some mums will have fairly quick and 'easy' births, while others will have longer ones. Some mums may also have their baby delivered by Caesarean section. Whatever the type of birth that lies ahead of you, the benefits of exercising will not be lost. You will recover better from any type of delivery if you are fit, healthy and well nourished.

Current research over the past ten years has shown that exercising through your pregnancy can bring about positive benefits and should not be detrimental to either the mother or the growing foetus. Two American gynaecologists – James F. Clapp III MD and Raul Artal MD – are mainly responsible for the most up-to-date research. Many of the references in this book are based on the research studies presented in James F. Clapp's book *Exercising Through Your Pregnancy*. James Clapp and his book have given us a greater insight into pregnancy and exercise, however there still remain many unanswered questions associated with exercise, pregnancy, delivery and the post-natal period.

'Women who exercise regularly during pregnancy maintain positive attitudes about themselves, their pregnancies, and their upcoming labour and delivery.'
James F. Clapp III MD, *Exercising Through Your Pregnancy*

Pregnancy and Fitness will help you understand the principles of safe and effective exercise during each stage of pregnancy, by enabling you to make informed decisions based on fact rather than old wives' tales. It will help you to exercise confidently throughout your pregnancy. And, while this book can't make the whole experience less intense or guarantee you an easy or quick delivery, it will help to keep you fit and healthy for the most wonderful physical challenge of a lifetime, and make sure you have the stamina needed to deal with the job of labour.

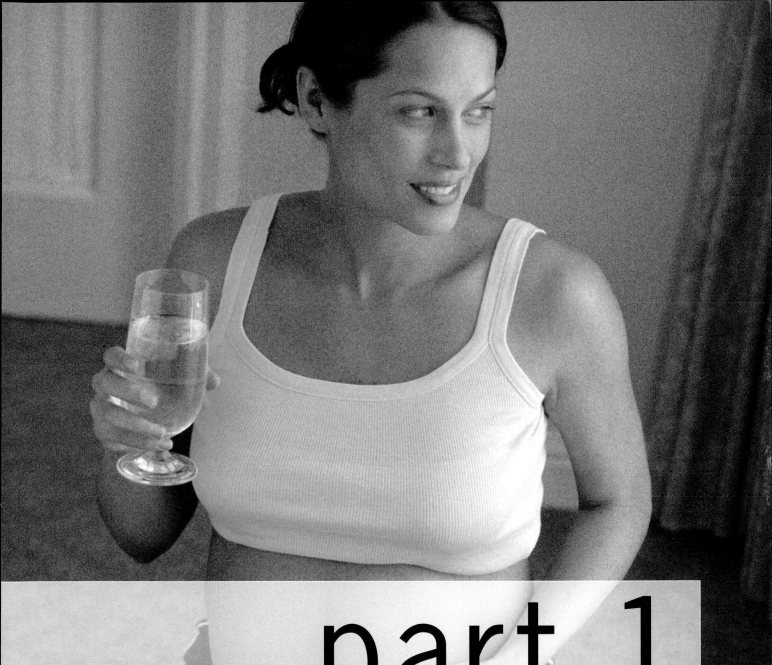

part 1
Your body during pregnancy

1. The three trimesters of pregnancy

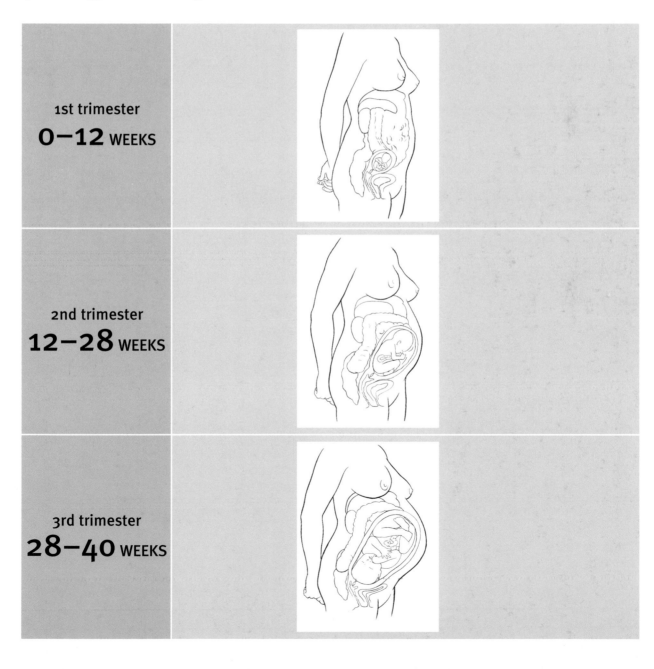

1st trimester
0–12 WEEKS

2nd trimester
12–28 WEEKS

3rd trimester
28–40 WEEKS

Remember that each pregnancy is individual. Some mothers-to-be will start to show quite early and some will have a neat little bump that doesn't show for ages. It's perfectly normal to compare yourself to other pregnant mums, as long as you remember that each and every one of you will carry your babies in a different way.

Your care team

Who wants a jack-of-all-trades and master of none? When I lecture around the country about pregnancy and exercise many people – members of the public and fitness professionals alike – ask questions like 'Why didn't my midwife know that?' and 'Why didn't my doctor know that?' Well the answer is a simple one: I can teach you how to exercise throughout your pregnancy, but I would not feel confident at all about facilitating the delivery of your baby. I know how to train your abdominals, but I wouldn't have a clue if your baby was too small for the date or you had a breach presentation. What is most important is the safe delivery of your unborn baby and your general health and well-being.

In an ideal world your medical care team will include experts in everything, but you may find that you have to seek medical advice from your medical and healthcare providers and fitness advice either from this book or a qualified pre-natal fitness instructor.

The antenatal care offered by healthcare providers will differ from person to person. Generally you will have an appointment to confirm and record your pregnancy. Prior to the 12th week of pregnancy (i.e. during the first trimester) you should have two appointments with either your doctor or midwife. You may then have appointments at weeks 16, 25, 28, 31, 34, 36, 38, 40 and 41 (the latter if you are overdue) of your pregnancy.

Remember ...

While you may come into contact with many fitness experts who are well qualified to deliver exercise in pregnancy, never forget that the last word should always go to the heath professionals involved in your care. *Always seek advice from your doctor, midwife or consultant if you have any concerns.* Your midwife is an expert and will often be the first point of contact with your healthcare team, so don't be afraid to ask for advice.

2. Advantages and disadvantages of exercise in pregnancy

Each pregnancy will be individual, so every mum-to-be will have her own aims in starting or continuing to exercise. This chapter provides you with general information about the good and bad points of exercising through pregnancy.

Advantages of exercising in pregnancy

- Possible reduction in back pain
- Improved core strength to support your spine and help you carry your baby around
- The correct type of exercise can prevent muscles from becoming over-tight and weak
- Improved posture
- Reduced likelihood of experiencing symptoms associated with pregnancy, such as leg cramps, swelling, constipation and varicose veins
- Improved circulation and blood flow
- Improved calcium absorption preventing future osteoporosis
- Time-out for mother, has a pampering effect and allows the mother to relate to the baby as she exercises
- Improved relaxation and possible improved sleep patterns
- Enhanced mental well-being, improved self-esteem and self-confidence
- Confidence in own ability to cope with labour
- Reduced chance of developing gestational diabetes
- Lower chance of high blood pressure
- Quicker recovery time after the birth
- Exercising helps curb excessive weight gain.

Research update

Research has shown that if you continue to perform regular weight-bearing exercise throughout your pregnancy (especially if you exercise right up to full term, if this is appropriate for you) this may have positive effects on your labour and delivery. It has also been suggested that pregnant women who exercise at least three times a week (for a minimum of 20 minutes at more than 50 per cent maximum heart rate each time) have significantly shorter labours than non-exercising women.

Unfortunately, exercising will not decrease the pain of labour, but it will allow muscles to be better equipped to carry out the task. It will also give you more of the stamina necessary to cope with pregnancy on a day-to-day basis.

Weight gain in pregnancy

Be aware that weight gain in pregnancy is not only normal it is a necessary and unavoidable aspect of carrying a baby. During pregnancy women tend to lay down fat in specific areas; again, the body has particular physical reasons for doing this. What we want to avoid in pregnancy, however, is excessive weight gain. Regular and sustained exercise in pregnancy can help play a part in controlling this. Exercising during pregnancy should never be about trying to keep your weight down – however, it can help you to avoid *excessive* weight gain.

Exercise and the placenta

Normal moderate exercise promotes the growth of the placenta and makes it more efficient in its ability to transport blood, nutrients and oxygen to your baby. This ensures that your baby still receives sufficient oxygen and blood supply even when you exercise. However, even when you are at rest this means that your baby can have a better supply of blood, oxygen and nutrients 24 hours a day seven days a week. It is also believed that this increased supply of oxygen may help protect the baby during labour and delivery. To maintain this benefit you should continue to exercise, as the placenta can decrease to normal size if you stop.

Exercise and your baby

When I was last pregnant, in 1996, it was thought that you should not exercise and raise your heart rate above 140 beats per minute (bpm). It was also thought that you should limit exercise sessions to 20–30 minutes. Part of the thinking behind this was the idea that if you exercise for longer than that, or push yourself harder, you may reduce the blood supply to the foetus, as your body would be busy sending blood and oxygen to your working muscles, heart and lungs. While this advice was well meant it was rather conservative.

More recent research has proved that when the mother-to-be is exercising moderately the blood supply to the foetus remains constant, and unless she exercises at a high intensity (over 80 per cent of her

---

Exercises that should not be attempted during pregnancy

- Deep-sea diving
- White-water rafting
- Diving
- Contact sports
- Horseback riding (due to risk of falling/being thrown)
- Skiing
- Water skiing
- Jet skiing
- Sky diving
- Exercising at altitude
- Gymnastics
- Surfing
- Ice skating
- Volleyball
- Basketball
- Squash
- Tennis

Note: if any activity becomes uncomfortable or just feels wrong then find an alternative type of exercise if possible rather than stopping completely, and take medical advice if necessary.

maximum heart rate or for more than 90 minutes) the supply to the foetus should not be compromised. For this reason a maximum heart rate of 70–75 per cent is now suggested, and a 30–60-minute cardio-vascular section. *Note, however, that these markers are only suitable for those who are already used to exercise.*

Disadvantages of exercising in pregnancy

- Possible over-exertion, which may contribute to general tiredness
- Possible increase in blood pressure
- Possible reduction in blood flow to the foetus if exercise is too intense or performed over excessive periods of time (see above)
- Possible increased chance of dips in blood sugar levels leading to hypoglycaemia
- Possible injury due to lax joints
- Possible stress on the pelvic floor with inappropriate exercises.

Can exercise be bad for your baby?

If you have what is known as a low-risk pregnancy then the answer is no, as long as you exercise safely and at a level that is appropriate for your stage of pregnancy. However, it is essential that you first get medical clearance to exercise once you know you are pregnant.

For those of you who may be new to exercise now is not the time to sign up for that 10 km run or to start mountain climbing! You can, however, start off slowly, look for specific pre-natal classes or ask gyms and suchlike if they have suitably qualified instructors to start you off on a beginner's programme that is suitable for someone who is pregnant.

3. Hormonal and physiological changes during pregnancy

Hormonal changes

Hormones are not just there to swim around your body and make you liable to extreme mood swings when you (or the people close to you) least expect it! They serve a very important purpose, and understanding them will help you to understand the physical and emotional changes that are taking place during this time.

Hormones very early in pregnancy are responsible for producing the signs and symptoms of child-bearing. The effects these hormones have will vary from person to person and with each pregnancy. The three main hormones that have physiological and emotional effect in pregnancy are oestrogen, progesterone and relaxin:

- **oestrogen** promotes growth
- **progesterone** relaxes smooth muscle tissue
- **relaxin** relaxes ligaments and fibrous tissue.

We will look at each of these in more detail below.

Oestrogen

Oestrogen is responsible for the growth of the uterus during pregnancy; during this time the uterus increases 1000 times in volume, up to a capacity of five litres. The smooth muscle in the uterus literally 'grows' during pregnancy. The uterus increases in weight from 45 grams to 480 grams. Initially the size of a small pear, it expands to that of a fair-size pumpkin (but not the same shape!).

Normal weight gain in pregnancy generally happens under the influence of oestrogen; this also has an effect on the way fat is distributed. Oestrogen is thought to prepare the muscular system for another hormone, called relaxin.

Initial effects of hormones

- Missed period
- Nausea and, in some cases, sickness
- Breast tenderness
- Tiredness
- Mood swings
- Urge to visit the toilet more frequently

Progesterone

The progesterone released during pregnancy will relax your smooth muscle tissue, including the gastrointestinal tract (stomach and intestines). Progesterone will increase your sensitivity to CO_2 causing you to feel out of breath more easily than you did before. During pregnancy the body works harder to get rid of CO_2 from your system, and so your rate of respiration increases.

Relaxin

Relaxin is perhaps the most important hormone in relation to exercising during pregnancy. It is produced very early in pregnancy, roughly just after the second week, and can stay in the system between five and six months after the delivery. It is also said that it may stay in the system longer when breast-feeding.

Relaxin is a hormone that is mainly responsible for relaxing ligaments and fibrous tissue in pregnancy. It does this so the body can prepare itself for carrying the baby and for labour. It relaxes the ligaments around the pelvis, allowing separation of the joints of the pelvis and therefore increasing space in the pelvis for childbirth. Relaxin works by increasing the amount of water in the connective tissue fibres (collagen) that make up our ligaments and tendons, allowing them to be more elastic. It also enables the abdominal muscles to stretch during pregnancy and the pelvic floor muscles to stretch during delivery. Relaxin has an effect on the whole body but specifically on the joints at the front and the back of the pelvis in preparation for the task of delivery ahead.

While this system is miraculous, it is also somewhat faulty as it not only affects the areas you need it to affect during pregnancy, but also gets to work on fibrous tissue throughout the body; the spine and knees, along with other joints, can also be affected. In pregnancy the walls of our veins can become affected. As we have more blood volume in pregnancy it is not uncommon for mums-to-be to experience varicose veins in the legs and even in the vulva.

The presence of relaxin is one of the main reasons that exercise needs to be specifically suited to pregnant women. As relaxin affects your body, you will become less stable around your joints. This has implications for the stretches and exercises you should do in pregnancy. Due to this lack of stability mums-to-be are more prone to injury during activity and less stable in their everyday movements.

Physiological changes

Pregnancy is a time of enormous physiological changes. If you are pregnant for the first time your body is probably changing and developing in ways that you never thought possible! The following pages will familiarise you with some of the major changes that you will experience, and how they can affect the way you exercise.

Breasts

Breast can often be tender and sore in the first stages of pregnancy. This may affect what exercise you can do in early pregnancy – for instance, you may find that it is uncomfortable to lie on your front to exercise. You may also find that you need to use a better support bra when taking part in any exercise. You may discover the cleavage you never had, without any accompanying increase in your abdominal area. However, while you may now have the figure you always wanted, you might be feeling too sick or tired to really enjoy it!

Throughout your pregnancy the weight and shape of your breasts will change. Fat is deposited in the breasts and milk-producing tissue is formed. All these changes are normal in pregnancy. Make sure you have your bra size measured at regular intervals by a professional who can also advise you which type of bra to wear when exercising, as well as on a day-to-day basis, and avoid wearing under-wired bras for exercise when you are pregnant.

Skin

During pregnancy the skin is affected by the hormonal changes within the body. Some of you may not notice any differences in your skin, while others will see marked changes. Have no fear: these skin changes generally disappear some time after delivery. You may find you get a narrow dark line down the middle of your abdomen, this is known as the linea negra. Some mums-to-be may get changes in pigmentation on the face, known as 'the mask of pregnancy'; using a sun block can help avoid this.

Stretch marks may also appear as the pregnancy progresses. These usually occur on the breasts and abdomen but can also occur on the hip and thigh areas. It really is down to luck and genetics as to whether or not you get stretch marks. Trying not to gain excessive weight in pregnancy can help. Although using specific pregnancy oils on areas prone to stretch marks has never been proven to help prevent them it is quite nice to pamper yourself in any case and, as long as the oils are safe to use in pregnancy, should not do any harm. Even better, make sure it's somebody else's job to gently massage pregnancy oils into your tummy or wherever else you fancy!

It is worth noting that these changes in the skin will not necessarily affect your exercise programme. However, one change that occurs will actually help you when exercising during pregnancy: the skin makes changes to help it deal more quickly and efficiently with increases in body temperature; pregnant women sweat more easily, which helps to dissipate unwanted heat as they exercise or go about their everyday lives.

Kidney and bladder changes

Pregnancy hormones and the growing uterus affect the bladder. You may feel that you need to urinate more often, especially in early and late pregnancy. This is normal so don't try to compensate by cutting down your fluid intake. In hot weather take care to exercise only moderately and make sure that you drink sufficient water.

Later in your pregnancy you may find that you naturally retain more fluid, causing swelling in the ankles, feet and legs. Exercise can help reduce this type of swelling by boosting circulation. When possible, elevate your legs, and avoid standing for long periods, or wearing clothing or shoes that are tight in one place. If you have an occupation that involves standing, or if you have an active lifestyle, you may find that special pregnancy support tights help – although they may not do much for your street cred!

Feeling bloated?

Water retention and swelling in the ankles, feet and legs during pregnancy is normal, but it is always worth mentioning to your medical care team if it is causing you any concern. Swelling around the hands and face is also common, but can occasionally indicate a problem, so do get this checked out.

Any swelling accompanied by blurred vision, a pain in your side and/or headaches must not be ignored, and you should seek medical attention as soon as possible.

Gabby's case study

Gabby used to take part in regular aerobic and conditioning classes before she became pregnant, as well as going on long walks regularly. However, from her 7th week of pregnancy she was so tired that when she arrived home from work she would have to eat and go straight to bed.

Gabby had to stop taking part in her regular exercise sessions as she was simply too exhausted. She did find that a brisk ten-minute walk at lunch helped to get her through the afternoon, but she couldn't manage any more.

The good news is that after 16 weeks of pregnancy Gabby started to have more energy in the evenings and was able to return to her normal exercise programme gradually for the rest of her pregnancy.

Many women find that they start to suffer from stress incontinence after giving birth – causing urine to leak out a little when laughing, coughing or working out, for example. This is perfectly common and wearing panty liners during exercise can make you feel a little more comfortable and confident. Doing the pelvic floor exercises on pages 43–4 regularly can really help in the long term.

Initial vascular under-fill

In the early stages of pregnancy, about the time the fertilised egg implants into the wall of the womb, hormones initiate reduced response and relaxation in blood vessels and muscle cells. This means that the heart, arteries and veins increase their elasticity and volume almost immediately. The effect of these changes means that for a short time there is not enough blood to circulate. Blood pressure will fall (this is called vascular under-fill) and you may often feel light-headed if you stand still for long periods or on standing up having been seated for some time. With this in mind, it's a good idea to avoid any sort of exercise in pregnancy that involves standing still or in one position for long periods of time. Think also about the transitions involved when getting up and sitting down. For instance, when exercising on the floor or a bench, turn on to your side and help yourself up with your arms. Performing an exercise or stretch in a seated, kneeling or all-fours position before standing up can help avoid feelings of dizziness and will also protect your abdominal area and joints.

If you are unfortunate enough to be severely affected by these symptoms you would be advised to rest and do only light walking or swimming until you feel well enough to restart your exercise programme. *Always consult your medical team if you feel unwell.*

These symptoms normally reduce or disappear by the 20th week of pregnancy. In some unfortunate mums-to-be, however, one or more symptoms may persist throughout the whole nine months. If you have to take a break from your exercise programme in early pregnancy due to severe symptoms of initial vascular under-fill you should return to exercise when feeling well enough, and only under medical guidance. On returning to exercise you need to start as a beginner and gradually rebuild your fitness level. It is important with any break from your normal exercise that you do not immediately return to the level and intensity of exercise at which you left off. The body loses fitness very quickly and will need time to regain and then maintain fitness levels.

Insulin

Insulin levels also increase during pregnancy and a small number of women will develop gestational diabetes mellitus. Symptoms of this are constant thirst and excessive urination. Gestational diabetes requires medical advice and control before you participate in any type of activity or exercise. The condition normally disappears after pregnancy.

Heart and circulation

When you become pregnant increased demand is suddenly placed on your heart and circulatory system. Your body is now supporting a growing baby as well as you and your increasing body weight. When exercising you are placing another demand on the system.

Gradually, the amount of circulating blood volume in the system increases. By the end of pregnancy you may have 40 per cent more circulating blood. Although there is an increase in red blood cells to carry more oxygen round the body, hormones from the heart and adrenal gland cause the body to hold on to more salt and water. This means that, although the volume of blood is increased, the increase in blood volume can be more from blood plasma than from red blood cell mass. At times this can increase feelings of tiredness and fatigue at various times of the day. It can also play a part in pregnancy anaemia, known as physiological anaemia.

Heart rate

To accommodate all these extra demands your overall blood volume will increase. Your heart chambers will expand, the amount of blood pumped per beat will increase and the amount of times the heart beats per minute can increase by up to 15 beats. This means that even if you are fit and healthy your resting heart rate will increase and exercise will elevate your heart rate quite quickly.

For this reason you will have to make adaptations to the length of time you exercise aerobically and, most importantly, you will need to gradually reduce the intensity of your cardiovascular workouts as your pregnancy progresses. You will also need to warm up very gradually and take time to cool down, as your heart rate will increase quickly and it will take longer for it to recover. These adaptations will be discussed more in the sections on cardiovascular exercise in Chapter 10.

If you wish to monitor the changes in your heart rate, you might consider investing in a heart rate monitor. However, I think this is probably an unnecessary expense and, in any case, I would not recommend that you rely solely on heart monitor readings during your pregnancy – a combination of other methods of assessing your heart rate (see pages 54–6) will probably be more helpful.

Respiration

Oxygen is essential to our everyday survival. During pregnancy the air you breathe flows through your system, eventually reaching your baby through the placenta and umbilical cord, ensuring that it receives sufficient oxygen to grow.

As already mentioned (page 9), progesterone increases your sensitivity to CO_2, causing your rate of respiration to increase. Simple tasks like walking up a flight of stairs may make you feel breathless. This does not mean that you are less fit than you were, it simply indicates that you are working harder and responding to changes in your respiratory system.

During pregnancy there is an increase in the basal metabolic rate; this in turn results in increased demand for oxygen. Towards the end of pregnancy there is a demand for up to 20 per cent more oxygen than was the case pre-pregnancy. In addition to the aforementioned increased sensitivity to CO_2, this means that breathing will become faster, and breathlessness is more likely as the body tries to expel increased levels of CO_2.

As the pregnancy progresses the size of the uterus increases and this eventually restricts the movement of the diaphragm. This can inhibit the ability of the diaphragm to contract fully and reduces the ability to take a full breath. This, combined with other changes to the respiratory system, increases the feeling of breathlessness. Under the influence of progesterone and relaxin, the body compensates for this problem by allowing the rib cage to flare, thus permitting the body to breathe in more effectively. These adaptations can often result in mild pain or discomfort around the ribs or mid-back. It is worth noting, however, that once the baby's head engages (drops into the pelvis) you may experience a wonderful sense of relief as your diaphragm is less restricted and it becomes easier to breathe.

Always breathe at your own rate and tempo, and warming up and cooling down gradually will help you to regulate your breathing – if you are unable to have a conversation while you are exercising then you are working too hard! Trying to breathe deeply or rapidly may cause you to hyperventilate. This can make you feel very dizzy, pale and clammy. If you do experience these symptoms, cup your hands over your mouth and nose and breathe normally until you recover.

'Beginning early in pregnancy, the increase in progesterone stimulates breathing, which improves the transfer of gases to and from the baby. It also makes women feel short of breath, but her lung function remains normal.'
James Clapp, *Exercising Through Your Pregnancy*

Core temperature

Your core temperature is the temperature of your body on the inside. Your foetus is always a little hotter than you are. Overheating, particularly in the very early stages of pregnancy, is dangerous for your baby. The foetus has no ability to get rid of heat so if you are hot your baby is hotter. Excessive increases in core temperature during very early pregnancy can cause birth defects. Later in your pregnancy excessive core temperature may cause the baby to be in distress. At the very worst you may become dehydrated which, when severe, can bring on premature labour. But please don't panic! We are not talking about you being warm enough to work up a bit of a sweat – and remember, too, that your wonderful body (particularly if you are already fairly fit and active) makes adaptations to your cooling system to prevent severe overheating. In simple terms, when you are pregnant your body is more effective at cooling your core temperature than when you are not pregnant. However you should still be alert to the problem of overheating, and take steps to avoid getting excessively hot.

Muscles and bones

As we have already seen, the hormone relaxin softens ligaments and cartilage. This means that your joints are less stable and more prone to injury. The lower back and hip joints can often become sore during pregnancy, particularly in the third trimester.

Such joint instability, along with weight change, can often affect posture. The changes in the centre of gravity that are experienced during pregnancy can cause an increased curve in the lumbar spine, known as 'increased lordosis'. They can also cause rounded shoulders, a condition known as 'increased kyphosis'. These changes in posture tend to make the chin jut forwards, and place stress on the neck and upper back.

Dos and don'ts of exercising in hot weather

Do wear loose, breathable clothing
Do drink plenty of water
Don't exercise in excessive heat
Don't wear sweatpants when exercising – shorts are better
Don't use hot tubs and saunas
Don't exercise when feeling unwell, especially if you have a temperature

---

Overheating Q&A

Q: I have been going to an advanced step class for some time now. I attended my last few classes before I knew I was pregnant. I worked really hard and got sweaty. Could I have harmed my baby?

A: As you were already used to step aerobics before you were pregnant it is highly unlikely. As you were already a regular exerciser, your body will have already developed an effective cooling system, and during pregnancy the body will be working to dissipate heat more effectively.

Another common postural change that can be caused by pregnancy is where the mum-to-be pushes her pelvis forwards, effectively 'hanging' on her ligaments, rather than using her muscles to maintain an upright position. This lazy posture is known as a 'sway back' and is often seen in adolescent males as well as pregnant women.

Any type of poor posture can place inappropriate loading on the joints and spine, causing backaches, headaches and muscle spasms. The Essential Core Stability workout on pages 35–41 will help you develop a good posture and avoid problems with posture.

Joints

Due to the effect of pregnancy hormones such as relaxin the joints can be unstable. Changes in the centre of gravity and weight distribution also contribute to incorrect posture and inappropriate loading on joints.

- Avoid exercises that go beyond the normal range of movement
- Avoid stretches that increase flexibility (normal-range stretches are fine)
- Avoid exercising in an unstable position
- Avoid overuse of one side of the body
- Avoid standing for long periods of time

When evaluating your exercises in terms of joint stability and suitability in pregnancy always think about the 'three Bs'.

1. Is the exercise *balanced*, does it give you a good base or is it unstable? Does the exercise overuse one side of the body or bring your body out of line?
2. Is your *back* in a safe position? Is the exercise suitable for your level of fitness and the stage of your pregnancy? Does the exercise cause stress on the back or pelvis?
3. Last but not least, *baby*. Does the exercise allow for the wonderful increasing girth of your abdomen and your increasing body weight, and are you able to get in to and out of the position comfortably?

Balance and changing centre of gravity

Due to the increasing size of your baby and the increased laxity in your joints, your centre of gravity will gradually change. Your body will not be as stable or balanced as it was previously. Exercise postures/positions need to be adapted to ensure that you are stable and the amount of balancing called for is minimal.

Round and broad ligaments

We have two main sets of ligaments that support the weight of the uterus. These are the round and the broad ligaments. The round ligaments are situated on either side of the uterus and attach to the front of the pelvis. The broad ligaments attach to the lumbar spine and the uterus sac. As pregnancy progresses, and the weight and size of the uterus increases, there may be some discomfort when performing activity. This may be felt around the groin area and on either side or in the lower abdomen, even as low as the vaginal area. The increased weight in the uterus can pull on the broad ligaments and cause pain in the lumbar spine and sacra iliac area. Regular core stability exercise can help prevent the pelvis moving too far out of position and over-stretching the broad ligaments. The wrong type of exercise, however, may increase movement in the pelvis and cause additional strain on the supporting ligaments.

Stomach and intestinal changes

Nausea and sickness are common in the first trimester, and these feelings are not just limited to mornings! Some mums-to-be continue to suffer from nausea right through pregnancy. It is worth noting that nausea during pregnancy is far worse on an empty stomach. Be aware that if you are often actually physically sick you must take care not to get dehydrated.

During pregnancy, hormonal changes cause activity in the stomach and intestines to slow down. Your digestion also slows, and the food you eat travels through your intestines slowly to promote better absorption of nutrients and the like (isn't that clever?). As your pregnancy progresses, your intestines and stomach will be moved upwards by the enlarging uterus and growing foetus. Unfortunately, these changes can bring about constipation, heartburn and indigestion. Drinking more water and exercising can help with the latter. I remember quite vividly that the only time I didn't feel sick in the first trimester of pregnancy, and a little beyond, was when I actually had food in my mouth or was doing some type of cardiovascular exercise. However, although I normally love garlic, tea, salads and fruit, I was not able to even smell any of these for quite some time without inducing nausea.

Avoiding that sick feeling

- Avoid letting your stomach get empty. Eat regularly and often.
- You may have previously eaten three well-balanced meals a day – now, however, such a gap between meals may be too much. Try having, say, five or six smaller meals throughout the day.
- Don't exercise on a full or empty stomach.
- Find out which foods will help you maintain blood sugar levels (see Part 4 of this book, on healthy eating during pregnancy).
- Ensure that you drink sufficient fluids: six to eight glasses per day.
- Try nibbling a ginger biscuit as this may help with sickness (just don't eat too many of them).
- Some say that smelling a lemon helps.

4. Safety considerations for exercising during pregnancy

Many of us are lucky enough to be blessed with a 'low risk' pregnancy – where there are no existing health concerns or difficulties – although you should always speak to your healthcare provider before embarking on any exercise programme. The accompanying box outlines some of the medical conditions that would mean you are not low risk, and therefore that general exercise may be unsuitable during your pregnancy.

Is yours a low-risk pregnancy?

Yours is **not** a 'low risk' pregnancy if any of the following apply.

- You have had three or more miscarriages
- There are hot, humid conditions, especially during the early stages of pregnancy
- You have a history of heart disease
- You have general poor health or medical problems such as diabetes, thyroid disease, kidney disorders and/or respiratory problems
- You have very low body fat (possibly due to ill-health or eating disorders)
- You are very overweight or obese
- You are on medication that alters cardiac output or blood flow distribution
- You suffer from anaemia
- You suffer from high blood pressure
- You have a history of premature labour
- Your medical team has confirmed that your baby is small
- You suffer from any injury or illness, such as problems with the nervous system, hip, back or joint problems
- You are expecting twins – if this is the case, extra caution is needed and specific programming essential

- You are suffering from symphysis pubic dysfunction (see the section about this on pages 163–4)
- You are experiencing any signs of labour or your waters have broken

If you have any of these conditions, you should not embark on a fitness programme without consulting your GP or midwife. Remember, your health may change during the course of your pregnancy, so be prepared to re-evaluate your fitness programme at any time.

Causes for concern

You should avoid exercise and seek medical advice if you suffer from any of the conditions listed in the accompanying box. Each of the points listed will require medical attention if it occurs.

Before you exercise

Before embarking on any exercise plan, make sure you consider the following points. Be honest with yourself!

- Do you have any medical problems with either this pregnancy, or have you had problems with any previous pregnancy?
- Was exercise a regular part of your life before you got pregnant, or are you relatively new to exercise?
- Are you being careful to adapt your exercise programme to your stage of pregnancy? This book will outline what you can and can't do at each stage of your pregnancy, but always listen to your own body.
- Are you feeling generally healthy and positive? Don't make yourself do any exercise just because you feel you should.

Remember that each pregnancy is different, and each mother will have different experiences of pregnancy. Every mum-to-be will cope differently, and will have different aches and pains. Each one of you will have a different pre-pregnancy fitness level and a different attitude towards exercise. *Pregnancy and Fitness* is not just about telling you what exercise you can and can't do – it is as much about learning to listen to your own body as anything else.

You can start new low-intensity activities if you are pregnant, but you should first seek medical or expert advice. Once you are pregnant, it is

---

Exercise should be stopped immediately if:

- you start to bleed
- you leak fluid
- you have pain down the front of your pelvis
- you feel dizzy, breathless or faint
- you feel strong pains in your abdomen
- you feel pain in your chest or numbness down your arm
- you can't feel you baby moving for long periods of time
- you see lights or 'floaters' in front of your eyes
- you get any sudden severe swelling
- you have severe or prolonged headaches

Now that you are pregnant avoid:

- strenuous exercise in hot, humid conditions
- exercising with an illness or high temperature
- exercising on rough ground, as your joints are more lax and prone to injury
- after the second trimester, weight-training exercises that involve raising both arms above the head

important that you think carefully before starting anything new. Be prepared to recognise any warning signs (see the box at the top of page 19), and make sure that you know what type of exercise is right for you: if exercise leaves you exhausted or in pain then it's not right. Tiredness can be a general symptom of pregnancy, but don't ignore excessive fatigue. Rest is as important as exercise and good nutrition.

You should have enough energy to attend to normal everyday activities and jobs, but if you find that you are excessively tired at the end of the day you may be doing too much. Cut down on your exercise programme for a few days and see if you recover. If you don't feel any better then your tiredness may just be due to your pregnancy – it is a hard job after all! However, if you do feel better after a rest then adjust your exercise programme to a more suitable level. Above all, be prepared to be flexible in your approach to exercise and change your fitness goals throughout your pregnancy.

Pre-pregnancy considerations

While this book is aimed at exercise during your pregnancy, for those of you who are not yet pregnant but are planning to be, the following information may be useful to you.

- Plan to get fit before getting pregnant.
- If possible, find a qualified pre- and post-natal fitness instructor to start you on a pre-pregnancy fitness programme (see the 'Useful addresses' section at the end of this book). It may also be worth asking your exercise instructor if they have read either this book or *Exercising Through Your Pregnancy*, by James Clapp, as this will help you to assess if their knowledge is up to date. If you do not have the luxury of an exercise instructor and you are starting a pre-pregnancy fitness programme alone, try to get a friend or partner involved as research has shown that you are more likely to stick to an exercise plan when working with a partner rather than alone.
- Consider diet and folic acid supplements.
- Avoid alcohol.
- Avoid smoking.
- Avoid use of recreational drugs.
- Avoid some prescription drugs (always check the label carefully and ask your GP or pharmacist for more information if necessary).
- Take adequate rest and relaxation.

Old wives' tales

Although the following statements are quite common, they have no basis in fact. Steer clear of taking too much notice of them.

'Exercise in pregnancy increases your risk of miscarriage.'
If yours is a low-risk pregnancy, then your chances of miscarriage are not increased by exercising. However, if you suffer from any of the conditions outlined earlier in this chapter (see page 18), you must seek medical advice before exercising.

'Exercise will cause your waters to break.'
Again, this is not the case. Your waters will break in due course, when the time is right.
'Exercise will take nutrients from your baby.'
If you are following a sensible, regular exercise routine that is comfortable for you then there is absolutely no reason why any nutrients will be diverted away from your growing baby. Of course, it is important to eat a healthy well-balanced diet, but that is true of any pregnancy – whether you exercise or not.

'Raising your arms over your head will wrap the baby's cord around its neck.'
'Exercise will make you go into labour prematurely.'
'Exercise will reduce blood supply to the foetus.'
'You must not exercise during the first 12 weeks of pregnancy.'
Again, none of these sayings has any basis in fact.

Miscarriage

If you are pregnant you are probably worried about the effects of exercise on your baby. Many exercise books will tell you that you should not exercise for the first 12 weeks of pregnancy. Indeed, you should avoid exercise during the first trimester if you are at risk of miscarriage – however, it is highly unlikely that exercise will either cause or contribute to a miscarriage. In fact, research has shown that the rate of miscarriage is actually lower in runners and aerobic dancers than it is in women who have stopped exercising or don't exercise at all.

Miscarriages are common during the first trimester – even before a pregnancy has been confirmed. Around a quarter of pregnancies result in miscarriage, and this is often accompanied by blame and grief. Early pregnancy can often bring about symptoms that may stop you from taking part in your normal exercise programme – you may be sick or suffer from severe fatigue. If this is the case, then it's quite OK to ease off on your exercise programme – you can always return to exercise when you feel well enough. However, when you do start exercising again, you should resume at a lower level than you were at when you stopped.

It is true that you are more at risk of miscarrying during the first trimester, specifically when implantation occurs. It is difficult to say exactly when this is likely to happen, as every woman is different, but if you are doing exercise that your body is used to it should not be an issue. If you are new to exercise and you start with a very light specific programme this shouldn't cause any problems either. I would therefore conclude that you should not stop exercising in the first trimester if you feel well enough and your medical care team think it's appropriate to continue. For instance, if you attend regular Pilates classes I believe that stopping this in the early stages of pregnancy would be a shame. You lose fitness very quickly and 12 weeks is quite a long time to go without exercise.

Even though miscarriage is a quite common occurrence in the early stages of pregnancy, medical advice should be obtained if you think you have miscarried. Vaginal bleeding or abdominal cramps are not normal in the second and third trimester and you should seek medical clearance before continuing with any exercise programme should either of these occur. Your medical team and healthcare providers should also check out any bleeding or abdominal cramps in the first trimester of pregnancy, although these may not necessarily be signs of any problems. Some women do experience warning signs in the early stages of pregnancy when they may have been due to have a period. Often, after investigation, everything turns out to be perfectly fine, however you should seek medical guidance immediately and avoid exercising until you are absolutely sure that everything is fine.

Please understand that, should you be unlucky enough to miscarry, it is very unlikely that anything you did contributed to it – it was not your fault!

5. The abdominal muscles during pregnancy

Your abdominal muscles provide a supportive muscular corset around the central part of your body, connecting your rib cage and pelvis, stabilising your spine and supporting your inner organs. As your baby grows they will also be called upon to accommodate the resulting extra weight and size. If you have strong and healthy abdominal muscles this will ensure that you can provide adequate support for yourself and your baby. First, however, you need to understand a little about each abdominal muscle.

Care of the abdominal muscles in pregnancy

As your baby grows your abdominal muscles need to stretch considerably to accommodate it. During pregnancy your waistline may increase by up to 20 inches, and the mid-line of your abdomen may increase from 11 inches up to 20 inches or more! In order to accommodate these changes not only must the muscles stretch, but the *linea alba* (see page 28–9) stretches and eventually separates in most women (this is known as *diastasis recti*). It is vital not to put undue strain on this area – it must simply be accepted that the abdominal muscles are weaker due to the stretching that is a natural part of pregnancy. This may lead you to ask 'Is abdominal training safe during pregnancy?'

The simple answer is that it is important to do certain abdominal exercises during pregnancy in order to help preserve correct posture and maintain as much control as possible over the abdominal area. If you have strong 'core stabilising' muscles this will help you to maintain correct pelvic alignment and avoid adopting a bad posture. Table 5.2 outlines what you can and can't do in terms of exercising your abdominals as your pregnancy progresses, and is based on a normal low-risk pregnancy. Please look back at the information on page 18–19 to ensure that yours is considered to be a 'low risk' pregnancy before embarking on any of these exercises.

The benefits of strong abdominal muscles during pregnancy

- Strong abdominals will support your back
- Strong abdominals will support the increasing weight of the baby
- Strong abdominals may assist the uterus when you are pushing your baby out
- Looking after your abdominals during pregnancy will make it easier to get them back in shape after delivery
- Strengthening the deep abdominals that work in conjunction with the pelvic floor will help prevent stress incontinence

Table 5.1 The main abdominal muscle groups

Name	Function	Diagram
Rectus abdominis	The *rectus abdominis* muscle is in two parts, which run down the front of the abdomen. The muscle fibres run vertically from the breastbone to the pubic bone. The muscle has three fibrous bands running across it, which can cause the chocolate-block effect that we know as a 'six-pack'. We all have these bands, it's just that some of us mere mortals never get to see them! This muscle also has a vertical fibrous band, called the *linea albi*, that splits it in the centre. It is this band that can separate in pregnancy as the baby develops – a process called diastasis recti – which happens to most women, but not all. **Function:** The rectus abdominis is mainly involved in flexion of the trunk – for example, when doing sit-ups, getting out of a low chair or sitting up from a lying position. **Note:** If this muscle is weak it may mean that you will suffer from bad posture – a condition that can worsen as your pregnancy develops and you carry more weight around on your front. Chapter 6 provides more information on postural changes in pregnancy.	
External obliques	These muscles run diagonally from the rib cage to the centre of the abdominal area, and fuse into the connective tissue and the pelvis on the same side as the ribs. These muscles tend to work alongside their opposite *internal* oblique muscles, as well as the rectus abdominis. The rectus abdominis and the external obliques have a limited effect on spinal stability, so are referred to as the 'superficial abdominals'. They should not be directly worked or stressed after approximately 12 weeks of pregnancy. **Function:** Working one side of the external oblique creates lateral flexion (sideways bending) and lateral rotation (twisting from side to side). Working both sides of the external oblique together assists in flexion of the trunk, during sit-ups or getting out of the bath, for example.	

Name	Function	Diagram
Internal obliques	These muscles run diagonally from the pelvis and the lower back to the lower ribs, attaching to the centre of the abdominal area and fusing into the connective tissue. These muscles tend to work alongside their opposite *external* oblique muscles, as well as the transversus abdominis. As the internal obliques and the transversus abdominis are the deeper muscles of the abdominals they have a huge effect on our spinal stability, and are referred to as the 'deep abdominals'. It is these two muscles that should be kept in good condition throughout pregnancy – they are vital to helping reduce back pain. **Function:** Working one side of the internal oblique creates lateral flexion (sideways bending) and lateral rotation (twisting from side to side). Working both sides of the internal oblique together assists in flexion of the trunk. The internal obliques also help to brace the trunk and expel things from the body – for example, when you sneeze.	
Transversus abdominis **(the 'corset muscle')**	The *transversus abdominis* is the deepest of the four muscles already mentioned. It wraps horizontally around the front of the torso and fuses into the connective tissue at the front of the abdominals. **Function:** The transversus abdominis supports the internal organs, and can contract to pull the tummy inwards towards the spine. The action of this muscle helps to stabilise the *linea alba* during abdominal actions. In pregnancy, it is important to work on this muscle as it can help to stabilise the linea alba when lifting, carrying and exercising, thus maintaining support for the spine. The transversus abdominis also helps to support the pelvic floor and is vital in creating core stability. If the transversus if weak, you are more likely to have back pain. This will mean that your back and abdominals will have limited support, and this may lead to discomfort as your baby gets bigger.	

Table 5.2 Advice on abdominal exercises in each trimester

Stage of pregnancy	General advice	Suggested activity
1st trimester **0–12** WEEKS	In an ideal world the abdominals should be in a good condition before a woman gets pregnant. If you are already doing exercise that involves the abdominals you can carry on as normal within the first 12 weeks of pregnancy. However, if you are having twins then you should start with the second-trimester exercises (see below). Always stop exercising if you are in pain or the exercises cause discomfort. There is no direct evidence to suggest that abdominal training is detrimental during these early stages – until approximately 12 weeks of pregnancy the foetus is contained within the pelvis, so it would be difficult to harm it through normal sit-up type exercises. However, common sense should prevail at all times. If it doesn't feel right then don't do it. If you are new to abdominal work when pregnant, move on to the second-trimester exercises.	Normal abdominal conditioning as long as this is not a new activity. Exercises that focus on correct abdominal hollowing will allow you to develop the necessary mind–body awareness and become skilled in this type of work. It is much easier to get to grips with this kind of training before the pregnancy starts to show and the abdominal muscles become stretched.
1st stage of the 2nd trimester **12–20** WEEKS	The foetus may now be out of the pelvis, so it is important to adapt the abdominal training from the first trimester. From approximately 12 weeks of pregnancy the linea alba may begin to split, particularly with second and subsequent pregnancies. Avoid sit-ups, reverse curls and oblique twists. Sit-up machines, back extension machines and rotation machines in the gym should also be avoided after 12 weeks.	Core stability exercises. The length of time for which the static contraction is held may need to be reduced, and, as always, it is important to encourage correct breathing. Pelvic tilts are also appropriate, both supine (lying), on all-fours and standing, as long as there is no evidence of increased diastasis (gap in the abdominal muscles). When performing pelvic tilts the abdominals should stay slightly contracted and there should be no doming of the abdominals (bulging outwards of the abdominals down the centre line of the tummy).

Stage of pregnancy	General advice	Suggested activity
2nd stage of the 2nd trimester 20–28 WEEKS	Due to supine hypotensive syndrome, supine lying needs to be adapted. This syndrome, if it is to occur, normally happens at approximately 20 weeks of pregnancy but can happen from 12 weeks. It is caused when the weight of the uterus impedes blood flow. This could lead to a feeling of light-headedness, nausea and, at worst, fainting. If you have any signs of supine hypotensive syndrome you should completely avoid lying on your back to exercise. If, however, you do not have any of the symptoms of this syndrome, then you can work on your back for very short periods – say, two minutes. A pillow or cushion may be used to prop you up when in a supine position. Pay special attention to avoiding any activity where the abdominals are seen to dome. You need to take care getting up from and down to the floor, and when changing position always contract the abdominals and use your arms to help you back to a seated position. Also avoid exercises that may put stress on the abdominal area, such as lifting heavy weights over the head. Be aware, too, that the action of getting in and out of some gym machines may cause you to get into a sit-up type position, which is not recommended at this stage of pregnancy.	Pelvic tilts on all-fours (avoid if suffering from carpal tunnel syndrome), standing pelvic tilts, lying-on-side pelvic tilts, hip-hitching on the side. Core stability work should be performed to enable the body to have sufficient endurance in the muscles that help maintain correct posture. This will at least lessen the chances of developing the back problems that affect nine out of ten pregnancies. Compared with earlier stages of pregnancy, you will need to reduce the length of time spent holding one position. Avoid pelvic tilts should a gap in the abdominals be present (see pages 28–9).
3rd trimester 28–40 WEEKS	At this stage it is far more likely that rectus muscles will split, if they have not already done so. This is due to the increasing size of the baby. It is also more likely that you will be affected by supine hypotensive syndrome. The rectus muscles will now be very stretched and therefore weaker than normal.	Core stability work held for shorter periods of time than in earlier trimesters. Pelvic tilts on all-fours (avoid if suffering from carpal tunnel syndrome), standing pelvic tilts, lying-on-side pelvic tilts, hip-hitching on the side. General trunk stability. Towards the end of the pregnancy the number of repetitions and the time spent doing pelvic tilts, hip-hitching and static abdominal work should be reduced. This is a very individual matter, however, and will depend upon the physical well-being of the mother-to-be, as well as her pre-pregnancy fitness and the size of the baby. Use alternative exercises that do not involve lying on your back.

Diastasis

As we have already seen, the rectus abdominis are two muscles that run down the front of the abdominals. They are joined in the centre by the linea alba. During pregnancy, when the linea alba is softened, it is stretched by the increasing size of the baby and the abdomen. This causes the muscles to stretch and weaken as they lengthen. Eventually the linea alba may split, and when this happens it is called 'diastasis'. The split tends to start around the belly button area and then moves upwards or downwards depending on how the mum-to-be affected is carrying her baby. The separation itself is not often painful as it is the connective tissue that joins the two sides of the abdominals that is actually moving apart. However, if the abdominals do part, this means that your back is not as well supported, your pelvis is less stable and your posture will change. While this is very common and will not cause a problem to your baby, it may cause you to experience back pain.

If you experience diastasis, it is important that you know how to manage the condition (doing the regular core stability exercises outlined on pages 35–41 will help you to condition your abdominals). Doing the wrong sort of abdominal exercise after 12 weeks, however, can exacerbate the problem of diastasis.

Testing for diastasis

While testing for diastasis is more appropriate in the post-natal period it can also be carried out during pregnancy to assess if diastasis has occurred. In any case, it is important that, after 12 weeks of pregnancy, you assume that you have diastasis or will have it, and avoid exercises that directly work or stress the rectus abdominis muscles.

The method

- Lie on your back supported by pillows (please don't do this test if you suffer from supine hypotensive syndrome – see pages 165–6) with your knees bent and your feet flat on the floor.
- Place the tips of your fingers down the centre of your abdominals below the belly button and press in and out a little to feel between the two halves of the muscle.
- Drop your chin slightly towards your chest and, as you breathe out, lift your head and shoulders off the ground.

- Feel for a separation between the muscles. You may be able to feel a slight dip even when the abdominals are normal, but there should be no gap or softness between the fingers.
- Repeat the test with your fingers above your belly button.
- If you can get more than two finger widths between the two sides of the rectus abdominis then diastasis has occurred.

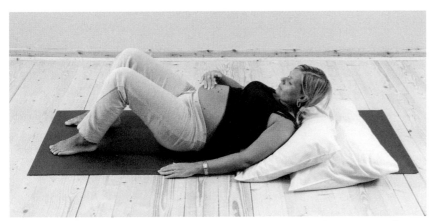

When you have completed the test, remember to bring your knees together and draw your abdominals towards your spine before you turn on to your side. Then use your arms to push yourself back into a sitting position before coming on to all-fours and slowly taking yourself into a standing position.

6. Core stability during pregnancy

During pregnancy as many as nine out of ten women suffer from back pain at some time, ranging from the mildly annoying through to the completely debilitating. So what can be done to combat this common condition? Core stability training is a good place to start.

Whatever other exercise you do during your pregnancy, you should ensure that you do some work to either improve or maintain your core stability. Not only can this help you to get your figure back after delivery, it may also help you to avoid back pain and maintain good posture throughout your pregnancy.

What is core stability?

Core stability focuses on strengthening your deep muscles, helping address the balance between overworked superficial muscles and the often neglected or under-used deep core muscles. Many people go to the gym and work out using fixed-weight machines, yet these machines allow you to sit or even strap yourself in so that you can work the muscles targeted in isolation, without having to focus on your core muscles to stabilise you. This is almost the direct opposite of the sorts of movement we do in everyday life – walking, lifting, running for the bus, carrying shopping – when our core muscles are working constantly to stabilise us without us even realising it. Machines in the gym can be great for toning up muscle, but they are of no help in improving your core strength.

  It is becoming more and more accepted that core stability can play a major part in helping improve the health and function of our backs during every-day life, so during pregnancy this type of activity is doubly essential. You need to address the way you walk, move, lift and bend to help protect against back pain. During pregnancy your changing weight distribution and centre of gravity combine with lax ligaments to considerably increase your chances of experiencing back pain. Incorrect posture and

Lack of core stability

Back pain is quite often experienced because the spine is not supported sufficiently by the muscles surrounding it, leaving it liable to 'wobble'. Core stability is not just about creating correct movement patterns and posture – it is also about using the deep core muscles to restrict excessive movement and so help prevent back pain.

weak core muscles increase the effect of poor weight distribution and place stress loading at different parts of the body, especially the spine. Work, stress, tiredness and simply being pregnant can all affect our posture and the tension present within our muscles. The discs between the vertebrae get nourishment from movement – so if our spine stays in the same position for long periods they aren't nourished sufficiently, and become dehydrated and stiff.

Approaching core stability

Consider building a house – it is vital to set good foundations. The house should be set on a solid base or it may easily collapse, subside or even fall down! Your body is very much the same. You can do exercises to strengthen or tone the muscles you can see in the mirror, but what about the muscles you can't see? In working your core muscles you are literally building your foundations, making your body not only toned but also stable and at less risk of injury. Who wants a body that may collapse, subside or fall over?

When doing core stability work for the first time it is essential to start with very simple, basic exercises to ensure that the correct muscles are being used. You should only progress when good technique has been achieved in these basic moves. The key to good core stability training is *quality before quantity* – please bear this in mind at all times.

As we have already seen, right from the start of your pregnancy special hormones relax your ligaments, which means that your joints, pelvis and spine become less stable than they are when you are not pregnant (see Chapter 3, on hormonal and physiological changes during pregnancy, particularly page 9). This can contribute to injury and pain. The ideal would be to develop your core stability before pregnancy, however it is not too late to start some form of core stability work once you are pregnant. It is important that the exercises you do are appropriate for you, your previous (non-pregnant) fitness level and the current stage of your pregnancy. Core stability is intrinsically linked with the principles of 'Modern Pilates', and many Modern Pilates teachers are specialists in exercises suitable for use during pregnancy. (You can use the information in the 'Useful addresses and websites' section at the back of the book if you want to find out more.) The stability ball exercises, and the Modern Pilates section in Chapter 16 focus on core stability.

Keep moving

If you are seated at a desk for a large part of your day, getting up out of your chair at regular intervals and moving around can reduce back and neck pain in pregnancy – as long as you take time to ensure that your posture is good! See pages 33–4 for more information on your posture during pregnancy.

Trunk stability

Throughout sections of this book we will not only refer to core stability, we will also use the phrase 'trunk stability'. This term incorporates core stability and also refers to shoulder and pelvic stability. In the introduction to core stability above, we talked about good posture and correct movement patterns for use in day-to-day activities such as walking and lifting – if we were to work on our core stability without correct shoulder and pelvic placement we would never be really effective in the way we move, lift and hold ourselves throughout the nine months of pregnancy and into the post-natal phase.

The main muscles involved in pelvic stability are the *gluteus medius* and the *gluteus maximus* (the latter has a stabilising effect on the pelvis, as well as being a 'movement muscle' and an important component in the bigger picture of back strength and support).

The lower body has to work harder as you gain weight and your centre of gravity changes. A strong gluteus maximus is important to help lift and move your beautiful increasing size. Therefore it is important that you do exercises that work your gluteus maximus muscles and help to condition the pelvic stabilising muscles and general muscles of the leg.

The *serratus anterior* and the *lower trapezius* have a stabilising function on the shoulder blades. Other muscles that play a part in upper back stability and posture are the *latissimus dorsi* and *shoulder retractors*.

The thoracolumbar fascia

The thoracolumbar fascia is a sheet of connective tissue covering the mid and lower back. The reason that I am introducing it at this point in the book is to help you to understand the reason why it is so important to use your core stabilising muscles.

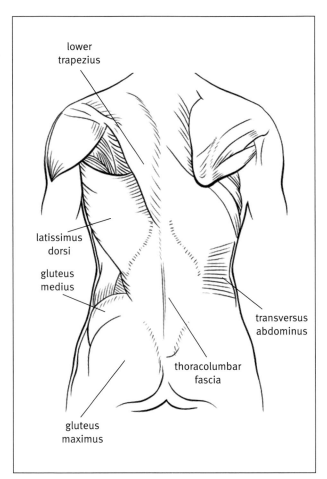

lower trapezius

latissimus dorsi

gluteus medius

transversus abdominus

thoracolumbar fascia

gluteus maximus

Main muscles used for trunk stability.

Think of the fascia being in the shape of a diamond. The lower trapezius pulls at the top of the fascia; the latissimus dorsi (see the muscle diagram on the previous page) pulls on the top sides of the fascia. The transversus abdominis and the internal obliques pull on the sides of the fascia, and the gluteus maximus pulls on the lower part of the fascia. When these muscles are all at optimum length and tone, they will all pull on the fascia when recruited, to tighten it and stop the spine collapsing.

The thoracolumbar fascia not only forms muscle attachments, it also creates a sheath through which the back extensors run. When we make bending-type movements, the gluteus maximus exerts a force that is transmitted through the fascia and helps tighten the back extensors within the fascia. This reaction allows the spine to stiffen, which is essential when doing things like lifting. It literally helps pull the back into a standing position.

Posture

During pregnancy, the increasing size and weight of your growing baby, changes to your centre of gravity, overworked abdominal muscles and less stable joints due to hormonal changes all conspire to leave your posture severely compromised. Your tummy may weigh you down at the front, exaggerating the curve of your lower back; the weight of your breasts may make your upper back rounded. Your body may try to overcompensate for these changes by making various adjustments, but they all mean one thing: bad posture. And bad posture may lead to the abdominals being stretched more than necessary, strain being placed on the lower and upper back, muscle tension in the neck, and even headaches. Towards the end of your pregnancy even walking may become difficult.

Due to your increasing size and changes to your centre of gravity, it will often be necessary for you to develop a stance that takes the position of your feet wider apart than usual, and this in turn will lead you to drop your hips from side to side, giving that typical pregnancy waddle. While this may look endearing at first, because the ligaments of your pelvis are relaxed, a waddling walk can end up giving you problems with your knees, hips and spine. Strengthening the buttocks and leg muscles can help maintain the stability of the pelvis and help you maintain good posture and walking technique. This may not be an easy task but be sure that your body will thank you in the end!

The importance of core stability exercises

If you do no other exercise while pregnant, at least make sure that you do some of the core stability or Pilates exercises featured in this book to help strengthen and tone the muscles that are attached to the thoracolumbar fascia. Not only will this help prevent back pain during your pregnancy, it will also help you maintain good posture and will undoubtedly help you get your muscles back in shape after delivery.

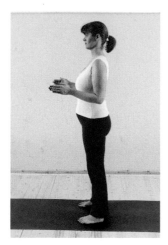

Good posture

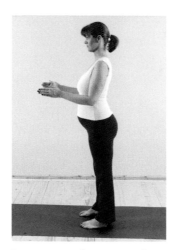

Poor posture (exaggerated curve in lower back)

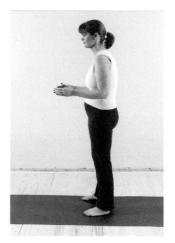

Poor posture (rounded upper back)

12 tips to help you achieve a better posture

1. Avoid sitting in low chairs
2. Avoid standing up for long periods of time
3. Remember to keep the back of your neck lengthened, with your chin dropped slightly towards your chest, and stand tall through your spine
4. Draw your shoulder blades down your back
5. Draw your abdominals slightly inwards
6. Keep your feet and knees hip distance apart (when possible)
7. Soften your knees slightly when standing still
8. Work your core stability muscles regularly
9. Strengthen your leg, buttock and upper-back muscles
10. Avoid bending over excessively
11. Wear good-quality supportive bras when exercising
12. Avoid high heels and very flat unsupported shoes

7. The essential core stability workout

The following sequence of exercises provides an essential workout for conditioning your core muscles, providing you with improved trunk stability and better positioning of the pelvis. It will work the deep muscles that are so essential to carrying yourself and your baby around as you get bigger.

This is a workout that you can complete three to four times a week as long as you feel comfortable doing so – it can also be combined with other types of exercise such as walking and your gym programme.

Basic exercises
Abdominal hollowing – standing
This is a basic exercise, and can be done at any time during your pregnancy.

Start position
- Stand with your feet hip width apart, and your knees ever so slightly bent (soft).
- Stand tall through your spine, with your sacrum (the triangle-shaped bone at the base of your spine) dropped towards the floor and not tilted upwards towards the ceiling.
- Keep the back of your neck lengthened, and your shoulders down away from your ears.

Action
- Breathe in to prepare, and feel your abdominals relax.
- As you breathe out, feel as if you are drawing your navel towards your spine.
- The gentle inward curve of your spine should remain the same throughout this movement.
- Breathing normally, hold your navel in for 3–6 seconds.
- Relax the position and move your feet.
- Repeat the exercise two or three times.

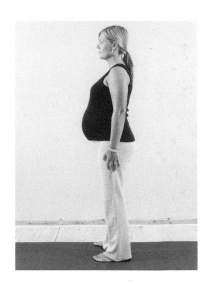

Hip hinge

This exercise is ideal throughout your pregnancy, but if at any time you experience back pain then stop doing this exercise and move on to the next one. Note that you will need a broom handle or similar sort of pole for this exercise.

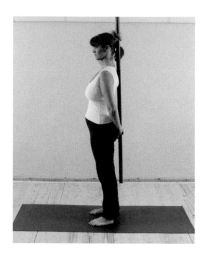

Start position

- Stand with your feet hip width apart, and your knees ever so slightly bent (soft).
- Stand tall through your spine, with your sacrum dropped towards the floor.
- Hold a pole behind your back, with one hand behind the top of your head and the other behind your buttocks.
- Breathe in to prepare.
- Breathe out, and as with the previous exercise, draw your navel in towards your spine.

Action

- Bend forwards from the hip, keeping your spine in line with the pole. Bend your knees lightly as you do so.
- Keep your shoulders drawn down your back and your tummy pulled in towards your spine.
- Push back up to the start position keeping your knees slightly bent. Your body weight should be even through both your feet.
- Start with five repetitions and then, once you have mastered the technique, you can build up to 15 repetitions.
- Note that the movement should not be held at the bottom. You should squat down and then come back up again – keep moving.

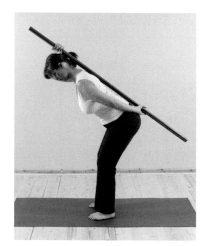

Tip

Your lower back should not change position as you contract your abdominals. There should be no movement in your pelvis, and your ribs should not lift up as you pull your navel towards your spine.

Abdominal hollowing – on all-fours (level 1)

This exercise is great for conditioning the core muscles around the abdominal area and back. It will also help stabilise the area around the sacroiliac joint, your pelvis and upper shoulder area.

Start position

- Kneel on all-fours, with your hands directly under your shoulders and your elbows slightly soft (not locked).
- Your knees should be directly under your hips, with the top of your feet flat on the floor if this is comfortable.
- Keep your spine lengthened and your neck in line with it (don't drop your head).
- Draw your shoulders down, away from your ears.

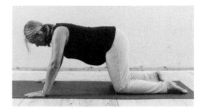

Action

- Breathe in to prepare.
- Breathe out and draw your navel towards your spine – remember to maintain the position of your spine – don't arch your back upwards.
- Breathing normally, keep your abdominals pulled in for up to 10 seconds.
- Relax back to a sitting position, to take the weight off your wrists, then repeat the exercise two or three times.

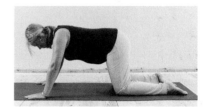

Abdominal hollowing – on all-fours (level 2 – cat 'pedals')

This exercise builds on the previous one. Make sure you are comfortable with level 1 before you move on to this one.

Tip

Your back should retain its natural curves during this exercise – don't over-arch your back inwards or keep it completely straight. Imagine a good standing posture, and translate it across to this exercise.

Start position

- Kneel on all-fours, with your hands directly under your shoulders and your elbows slightly soft (not locked).
- Your knees should be directly under your hips, with the top of your feet flat on the floor if this is comfortable.
- Keep your spine lengthened and your neck in line with it (don't drop your head).
- Draw your shoulders down, away from your ears.

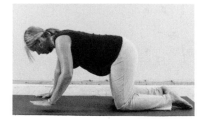

Action

- Breathe in to prepare.
- Breathe out, and draw your navel towards your spine.
- Keeping your abdominals hollowed and the position of your spine stable, lift one hand off the floor, keeping the elbow of your 'balancing arm' soft.
- Breathe normally and hold this position for a few seconds, keeping your body as still as possible.
- Lower your hand to the floor and repeat the movement on the opposite side (almost like a very slow pedalling motion as you move from one side to the other, but made with your arms, rather than your feet – a bit like a cat 'padding' its front paws, hence the title of this exercise).
- Repeat three or four times on each side, keeping your abdominals hollowed and your shoulders pulled down and away from your ears.

Tip

Throughout this movement concentrate on keeping your trunk stable – don't rock from side to side.

Abdominal hollowing – on all-fours (level 3 – knee lifts)

This exercise builds on the level 2 version, above. Make sure you have mastered levels 1 and 2 before you move on to this one.

Start position

- The start position is exactly the same as the previous exercise.

Action

- Breathe in to prepare.
- Breathe out, and draw your navel towards your spine.
- Keeping your abdominals hollowed and the position of your spine stable, lift your right knee off the floor slightly – no more than 1 inch.
- Keep your knee in line with your hip, and keep your foot on the floor. Your lower body will shift slightly, but avoid twisting the lower body or dropping the supporting hip down to one side.
- Breathe normally and hold this position for a few seconds, keeping your body as still as possible.
- Lower your knee to the floor and repeat the movement on the opposite side.
- Repeat three or four times on each side, keeping your abdominals hollowed and your shoulders pulled down and away from your ears.
- You can develop this exercise by lifting your knee and your hand on the opposite side at the same time.

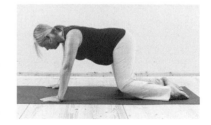

Stability ball work

Hip hinge on the stability ball

This exercise is great for strengthening your thighs and core stability muscles.

Start position

- Sit upright on the stability ball, with your feet hip width apart.
- Keep your spine and the back of your neck lengthened – don't slouch.
- Cross your arms over your chest.

Action

- Breathe in to prepare.
- Breathe out, drawing your navel towards your spine and lean forwards 3–6 inches, initiating the move from your hips not your spine.
- Exhale as you return to your upright seated position.
- As you lean forwards feel the sensation of your spine lengthening and your weight shifting into your legs.
- Repeat this movement.

Choosing a ball that is suitable for your height

- If you are under 5 foot 8 inches tall then you will need a 55 cm stability ball.
- If you are 5 foot 8 inches or over, then you will need a 65 cm stability ball.
- NB: Your bottom should not be lower than your knees.

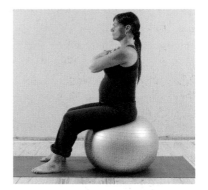

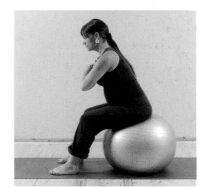

Tip

If you are not sure that you are keeping your abdominals hollow throughout this movement, try the following: place just one arm across your chest, and place two fingers of the opposite hand on your belly button; as you lean forwards into the movement you should still feel that your abdominals are contracted – not bulging out towards your fingers; if this does happen spend some more time working on the first abdominal hollowing exercise in this section; make sure you can get that one right before you move on.

Foot lift

This exercise is suitable for keeping the muscles that help stabilise the pelvis toned, and improving the circulation in your legs.

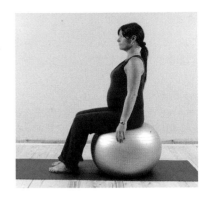

Start position
- Sit upright on the stability ball, with your feet hip width apart.
- Keep your spine and the back of your neck lengthened – don't slouch.
- Keep your hands on the side of the ball.

Action
- Breathe in to prepare.
- Breathe out, drawing your navel towards your spine and lift one heel, then the whole foot, about an inch off the floor.
- Breathing normally, hold this position for a few seconds and then lower the foot to the ground.
- Keeping your weight evenly distributed and your abdominals hollowed, change feet and repeat on the other side.
- Start with four lifts alternating between both feet (two on each side), and build up so that you repeat the exercise several times.

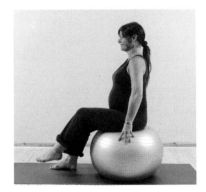

Tip

Once you have tried a couple of lifts on either foot you may find it easier to take your hands off the ball and out to the side to maintain your balance. If you start to wobble too much then place both feet on the floor and put your hands back on the ball.

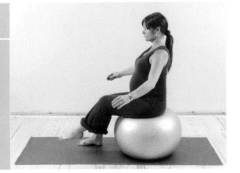

Reverse bridging

This exercise is suitable for use in the first two trimesters. It will strengthen your legs, buttock and core stability muscles.

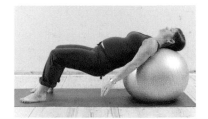

Start position

- Sit on the stability ball and gradually walk your feet away until the ball is resting between your shoulder blades and the neck is supported in a flat position.
- Keep your knees bent and your feet directly under your knees, hip width apart.
- Drop your arms down to the side.
- Drop your buttocks and lower your ribs down towards the floor.

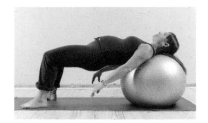

Action

- Breathe in to prepare.
- Breathe out and draw your navel towards your spine.
- Slowly lift your hips and ribs until they are in line with your shoulders, then hold.
- Lower slowly to the start position and repeat.
- Start with three repetitions and build up to 10–15 repetitions.

Intermediate

- Repeat the above exercise but with your arms resting across your chest.
- Try lifting alternate heels off the floor.
- Hold the lifted position and take both arms up towards the ceiling until your palms face each other (shoulder width apart), take one arm back in line with the forehead, the other arm by the side of your body, then bring your arms back to the centre. Switch arms and repeat several times on each side.

Tip

Your weight should be supported through the shoulder area and you should avoid moving your body backwards and forwards – the ball should stay still while your body moves up and down. Avoid over-arching your back at the top of the movement and ensure that your ribs stay in a straight line with your hips. Get someone to hold the ball until you are used to this exercise.

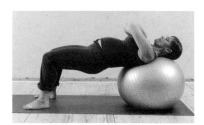

8. All about the pelvic floor

Your pelvic floor provides an essential support for your growing baby during pregnancy. This chapter gives you all the information and exercises you need to achieve strong and healthy pelvic floor muscles.

What is the pelvic floor?

The pelvic floor is composed of an essential group of muscles that are quite often overlooked. It acts like a strong, muscular hammock between your legs. Your pelvic floor helps to keep all your internal organs (including your uterus) in place; it allows the bladder to function effectively, and it helps you to control your bowels; not only that but, in the long term, exercising the pelvic floor muscles can help to improve your sex life – although I understand that this is probably not your primary concern at the moment! For these reasons, you should do pelvic floor exercises daily, not just during your pregnancy but for the rest of your life.

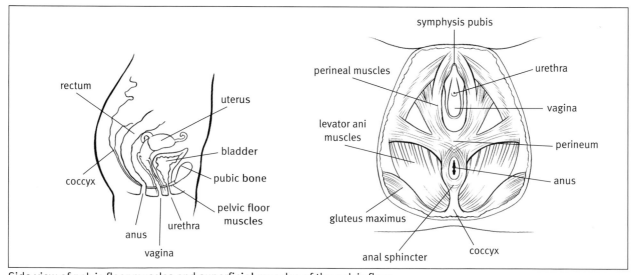

Side view of pelvic floor muscles and superficial muscles of the pelvic floor

The pelvic floor is made up of both deep and superficial muscles that are attached to the pubic bone at the front of the pelvis, the coccyx at the end of the spine and the 'sitting bones' at the bottom of your pelvis. Your urethra, vagina and rectum all pass through the pelvic floor.

Finding your pelvic floor

There is an easy way to feel the action of your pelvic floor muscles and you can try it next time you visit the toilet. By stopping your urine flow, holding for a second or two, and then restarting it you are using your pelvic floor – and this is a good indication that the muscles are working correctly. This should not be done as a regular exercise, however, as doing it too frequently may make you more susceptible to bladder infections. There are far more effective ways to work on your pelvic floor, as we shall see.

Why should I exercise my pelvic floor?

Pregnancy and childbirth have a weakening effect on the pelvic floor. Even if you do not have a vaginal delivery you may still experience weakened pelvic floor muscles due to the weight of the baby during pregnancy and the resulting increased pressure on the pelvic floor. During pregnancy the pelvic floor is stressed, and this means that, unless you exercise it, it will not be as strong after delivery as it was before you gave birth.

Pelvic floor exercises will help prevent weak pelvic floor muscles after childbirth. It is quite common for women to experience stress *incontinence* (where a little fluid is leaked when coughing, laughing or exercising, for example) towards the end of a pregnancy and after childbirth. If this is something that you are experiencing then pelvic floor exercises are just the thing for you. Even if your pelvic floor muscles are working well, keeping them strong is very important.

Pelvic floor exercises

There are many ways to exercise your pelvic floor. Below I have described some of the most effective ones. Please bear in mind that the pelvic floor muscles can be exercised every day, unlike other muscles, which need 'rest days'. You don't need to overdo it – a few minutes, several times a day is sufficient. Don't feel bad about having days when

---

Correct form for pelvic floor exercises

Many people do pelvic floor exercises incorrectly. You should avoid:

- actively contracting the abdominals
- gripping with the muscles of the legs
- tensing or clenching your buttocks
- holding your breath as you work your pelvic floor
- tensing your shoulders (you also need to keep your hands relaxed).

Research update

Research has shown that women who follow an eight-week programme of pelvic floor exercises during their pregnancy have less urine leakage than women who do no exercises. This finding persists, even a year after the birth.

you don't do them, but do try to stay focused and keep doing them regularly. After all, the time you need to spend on them each day is minimal when you think of the rewards.

Table 8.1 Pelvic floor exercise routine

1	• Breathe normally and sit or stand upright. • Without visibly moving, imagine that you are pulling your vagina, then urethra and then back passage, upwards, and feel the sensation of them lifting towards your belly button. • Hold this position and then slowly release. • Work towards holding the contraction for 10 seconds, although it may take some time before you can achieve this. • Repeat this exercise several times a day.
2	• Follow the same steps as above, but this time don't hold the contraction – contract and release the muscles in a fast 'pumping' action. Imagine you are switching a light on and off. • Repeat this 10–15 times.
3	• Sit on a chair, toilet or stability ball. • Perform the pelvic floor exercises as before, hold for a few seconds and then release slowly. • Now place your elbows on your knees and lean forwards. Repeat the same pelvic floor exercise again, but this time notice that you can feel the movement more around your urethra and vagina, and less around your back passage. • By alternating between sitting upright and leaning forwards, you are able to isolate different areas of the pelvic floor.
4	• Think of the pubic bone at the front of the pelvis and the coccyx (at the tail end of the spine) at the back of the pelvis. • Imagine drawing these two parts closer together, hold for up to 10 seconds then slowly relax the muscles. • Focus on the 'sitting bones' at the bottom of your pelvis. Think of drawing these two points closer together, again hold for up to 10 seconds and then relax. • Now think of the front, back and bottom points all drawing closer together. Feel as if you are pulling these muscles up towards your belly button. Hold for up to 10 seconds and then slowly relax.
5	• Lift your pelvic floor upwards as described in the previous exercise. • Imagine a lift going up and down – hold your pelvic floor muscles at each level, trying to reach five levels. • Release your pelvic floor muscles slowly, again stopping at each level on the way down.

If you are already having pelvic floor problems all is not lost! You should see your GP and ask for referral to the continence nurse (a physiotherapist who specialises in women's health). Alternatively, contact the Continence Foundation (see the 'Useful addresses and websites' section at the end of the book).

I understand that this book is not about exercising after your pregnancy, however I want to share the following facts with you. Not only are they interesting, they are also a great incentive to start doing pelvic floor exercises right now, regularly and often.

- One out of four women over 40 have some type of stress incontinence.
- One in 20 women still have severe stress incontinence three months after giving birth. (We often think of a weak pelvic floor meaning that you leak a little urine when you jump, cough or sneeze, during pregnancy, but many women find they can't ever run again after having children without a small amount of urine leaking out. This is 'permanent' stress incontinence, although mild.)
- You can become rectally incontinent after delivery. (Lovely thought!)

Can I make my pelvic floor too strong?

Some women may have concerns that they can exercise their pelvic floor too much, and that it will become too strong and thus hamper delivery. This will not happen! It is a misconception that has been aided in years past by women being told that their pelvic floor and abdominals were too strong in labour and that they wouldn't stretch to allow the baby to be delivered. A strong muscle is more able to stretch than a weak one. It is also more likely to return back to its normal shape. Recent research has shown that women who exercise their pelvic floor muscles very regularly often have shorter second stage labours.

Jane's case study

Jane is a regular exerciser of slim build. Her first baby was quite big and although she had a normal vaginal delivery, pregnancy and birth left her pelvic floor severely weakened.

By doing regular pelvic floor exercises, Jane has really improved the strength of her pelvic floor and has no real problems with her bladder. However, she does find that she can't run more than five miles without desperately needing to go to the toilet, and doctors have advised her that without surgery this is likely to remain the case.

However, as long as Jane keeps exercising her pelvic floor her condition will not get any worse, and there will be no need for her to undergo surgery. As a result she keeps her weight under control, avoids excessive high-impact running or running in excess of five miles. She works on her pelvic floor exercises every day and takes a regular Pilates class to help condition her core stability muscles.

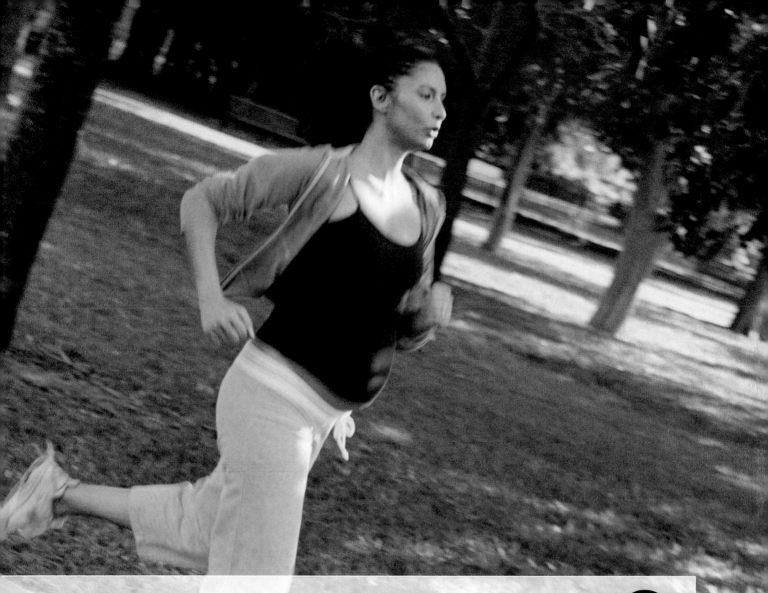

part 2

Cardiovascular exercise and fitness
programmes during pregnancy

9. Exercise basics

We have already talked about the physical changes you will experience during pregnancy. This part of the book will look in more detail at the practicalities of incorporating exercise into your everyday life during pregnancy. Make sure you are clear on the exercise basics contained in this chapter before you proceed – they will provide you with all the information that you need to be aware of before you get started.

The effects of exercise

During exercise there will be increased demand for blood to be pumped into your heart, lungs and working muscles – this demand *will not* reduce the flow of blood and oxygen to your baby as long as the exercise is not excessive, or for prolonged periods of time (over 90 minutes). As already mentioned (page 13), during pregnancy your blood volume increases by up to 45 per cent, and with it the amount of oxygen in your body. Regular exercise can also increase blood volume up to an additional 10 per cent. These increases in blood volume mean that you and your baby have a more than sufficient blood supply – so there is no need to worry about reduced blood supply to your baby as you exercise.

Other effects of exercise on the baby

In the Victorian era pregnant women were encouraged to stop doing even the most basic tasks. In the twenty-first century we have a much better informed approach to exercise and pregnancy.

Popular misconceptions about exercise and pregnancy explained

Many pregnant women have misconceptions about exercise that have been handed down through the generations. While this is understandable, many of these have now been proved wrong. We will now have a look at some of the more popular misconceptions.

Cardiovascular exercise (specifically step aerobics) in early pregnancy can cause your core temperature to rise

During pregnancy it is never advisable to get overheated, but from early pregnancy, as explained earlier, your body will make adaptations to get rid of any excessive heat. This is your body's way of coping with excess heat now that you are pregnant – it is as if you have your own inbuilt thermostat that will regulate your body temperature efficiently and enable you to dissipate any excess heat created as you exercise, so 'internal overheating' will not be a problem.

You should always observe the following guidelines, however.

- **Don't** do cardiovascular exercise in excessive heat.
- **Don't** exercise above level 7 of the rate of perceived exertion (RPE) shown on pages 55–6.
- **Don't** exercise if you are unwell or already have temperature.
- **Don't** start high intensity cardiovascular exercise if you were unaccustomed to it pre-pregnancy.
- **Do** make sure you drink sufficient fluids throughout your exercise session.

It is also worth noting that exercising in water dissipates body heat more easily, thus helping you to keep cool. However, when you get out of the water you may feel a little more hot and uncomfortable when trying to get dry and dressed – presuming you are even able to squeeze into a changing cubicle!

Cardiovascular exercise that involves some impact causes the waters to break

Unless your waters are due to break, aerobic exercise should not cause them to do so prematurely. Mums-to-be who are regular runners can run comfortably throughout their pregnancy without any risk of this happening. However, it is advisable that you do not start any jumping or running activities in pregnancy if you did not do them beforehand.

Cardiovascular exercise will divert the blood supply away from the baby and into the mum-to-be's muscles, heart and lungs instead

As I have already emphasised, regular moderate exercise does not divert blood supply, oxygen or nutrients away from your baby. Rather, it promotes the growth of the placenta and makes it more efficient in its ability to transport blood, nutrients and oxygen to the baby. This ensures that your baby still receives sufficient oxygen and blood supply even when you exercise. If the placenta is encouraged to grow in this way, then even when you are at rest your baby will have a better supply of blood, oxygen and nutrients 24 hours a day, seven days a week. It is also believed that this increased supply of oxygen may help protect the baby during labour and birth. However, as I also mentioned earlier, in order to maintain this benefit you should continue to exercise as the placenta can decrease to normal size if you stop exercising for any sustained period of time.

Cardiovascular exercise will divert nutrients away from the baby as the mother-to-be will be using them as 'fuel', and this may cause the baby's development to be restricted

The higher blood volume during pregnancy also provides additional protection for the supply of nutrients to the baby. As mentioned above, exercise will in fact increase the efficiency of the placenta during pregnancy and will not only help to maintain oxygen supply to the baby while you exercise, but will also help foster a good nutritional supply.

It is important, however, to eat sufficiently during your pregnancy. While this is true whether you exercise or not, you will benefit from knowing about nutrition if you are active. Not only will you get more from your workouts, but you will also avoid the unnecessary fatigue that can result from not eating the right types of food.

Cardiovascular exercise can cause the baby's heart rate to drop or increase too much

Exercising for approximately 10 minutes will mean that your baby's heart rate will rise. As you continue to exercise, your baby's heart rate will get faster, and once you have stopped exercising it may stay elevated for up to 15 minutes before returning to normal – but it will eventually return to normal. Very strenuous exercise may cause the baby's heart rate to stay

Research update

Research has shown that babies born to exercising mums tend to be 'fitter' and get higher scores in general health tests at birth. They also seem to be able to deal with stress better, which can only be a good thing when you are thrust into a brand new world from a nice warm womb!

Keep moving

Research has shown that women who exercise regularly and then give up in the last few months of pregnancy put on weight at the same rate as non-exercising women; this means that their babies will quickly lose the benefits of their formerly healthy approach to life.

For you and your baby to gain benefits from exercise you can continue with some type of training (even if this is just in the form of light walking or swimming) right up to the end of your pregnancy, as long as you are feeling well and don't have any medical conditions. You will obviously need to adjust your exercise programme as your pregnancy progresses, but hopefully the health benefits it offers will motivate you enough to keep your walking boots on!

elevated for up to 30 minutes after you have stopped, and this is one reason the American Council of Obstetricians and Gynaecologists (ACOG) recommend only exercising to 70–75 per cent of your maximum heart rate when pregnant.

It is important, though, to understand that these heart rate changes are a normal response to exercise and do not cause the baby distress or affect normal foetal behavioural/development patterns.

Heart rate increases in a baby can also, however, be due to changed stress or adrenalin levels in the mum-to-be, which is not such a positive thing. However, this is most definitely not the case when you exercise – on the contrary, exercise is a completely positive way to elevate your baby's heart rate.

Exercise can cause miscarriage

Research has found that mums who exercise regularly throughout pregnancy are less likely to have complications during pregnancy and delivery than their sedentary counterparts. So, in fact, the opposite is true: mums-to-be who exercise are less likely to miscarry.

Aerobic exercise (including running or aerobic dance in early pregnancy) has not been shown to increase or decrease the rate of miscarriage.

What to do when you are pregnant and new to exercise

First of all, you must visit your GP to get medical clearance to exercise. If you get the go-ahead, be realistic. You may feel excited and energised and ready to leap for joy, but now is not the time to enter a 10 k race!

Start with a walking programme (see page 79) and begin regular pelvic floor and core stability exercises (see pages 35–41 and 43–4). Also work on stretches for the hip flexors, hamstrings and chest muscles (pages 139–42) to balance your programme. Aim to do three minutes' gentle stretching, building up to 5–10 minutes as you progress.

There are no short-cuts so start off slowly and gradually. Exercise during pregnancy should be seen as a way of staying fit and healthy and providing the best environment you can for your growing baby. It should not be used as a method of losing weight or stopping yourself from changing shape. Take care of yourself like never before but be proud of your changing shape too.

Two's company

You may find that it helps to enlist a friend or partner to start this gentle exercise programme with you. A fellow pregnant friend would be wonderful; however, a partner who is a bit of a couch potato could be just as useful – after all, looking after a baby is not a job for the faint-hearted, and both parents are likely to benefit from being fitter. Even an enthusiastic grandparent-to-be may fit the bill nicely!

What to do when you are pregnant and a competitive athlete

If you are a competitive athlete or exercise teacher you probably already have a high level of fitness. Pregnancy is not the time to improve on this. You will probably continue to exercise at a higher level than most average pregnant women, but you will need to make adaptations to your existing training programme throughout your pregnancy. It is important that competitions are put on hold, and world records will have to wait. You will be able to train through your pregnancy at relatively high levels as your muscles, joints and cardio respiratory system will already be stronger and better developed than most. However, it is essential that your medical care team knows of your intentions and is happy to support and advise you though this.

You should gradually reduce both the intensity and length of your training periods as your pregnancy progresses, specifically after the 20th week. As long as you feel fine, the baby is developing well and your medical care team is happy with the overall picture, however, there is no reason why you cannot carry on exercising at a modified level until you give birth.

During your pregnancy you need to eat and rest sufficiently for your developing baby. When you are pregnant you need approximately 300 calories per day on top of your normal daily allowance; exercise super-imposes extra demands on top of this. Those of you who exercise and have fairly active lifestyles may need up to 500 extra calories per day. If you exercise more intensely or for more than 10 hours per week, you may need up to an extra 600–800 calories per day.

How do I know if I am doing too much exercise?

Pregnancy brings its own needs and it is not unusual for you to feel more tired than usual. However, you should have enough energy to go about your normal daily activities. If you haven't, ask yourself if you are doing too much exercise? Are you getting enough rest? Are you eating and drinking sufficient fluids? You need to readdress all these questions and adjust your exercise programme as necessary, or up your rest and nutrition. Eat sufficient calories to support you, your baby and the extra energy requirements you need in order to be able to exercise.

Dos and don'ts of working out

- **Do** stop if you feel light-headed, very tired or very hot.
- **Do** drink plenty of fluids before, during and after exercise – small regular sips are best.
- **Do** visit the toilet as often as you need to.
- **Do** wear a sports bra and good training shoes.
- **Don't** exercise so hard that you are unable to hold a conversation.

Ways to measure how hard you are working (exercise intensity)

- Heart rate monitoring
- Talk test
- Rate of perceived exertion
- Post-workout fatigue

Your baby should move at least twice in the 30 minutes following your exercise programme. Monitor this and if this doesn't happen regularly then check with your medical care providers and modify your exercise programme as necessary. Most of you will find that after your exercise session you sit down for a well-earned rest and a drink, perhaps a chat with friends, and then baby decides to do its own aerobic session. Didn't they tell you that babies are experts at in-womb kick-boxing?

As I mentioned, I taught fitness classes throughout all my pregnancies. I can't say I monitored my babies' movements religiously within the 30 minutes following exercise as I was normally too busy chatting with my class members while propping up the bar (soft drinks only, of course). However, I often returned home, looking forward to putting my feet up for a while, and my baby would get its revenge – not comfortable physically, but it was good to know that my baby was well and active, and not too tired after all my teaching.

Monitor how hard you are working

There are many ways of monitoring how hard you are working (your 'exercise intensity'). If you monitor certain things when you are exercising (see the accompanying box) you can actually measure how hard your heart is working, which is essential to make sure you are not overdoing it.

Although most of the methods listed in the box are usually reasonably accurate, when you are pregnant they become less accurate and have to be adapted. Never fear, though – with some common sense and a little know-how they can still be a useful tool in measuring your level of exertion.

Heart rate monitoring

In 1994 the original ACOG (American College of Obstetricians and Gynaecologists) stated that you should not exceed 140 beats per minute (bpm) when exercising aerobically. This recommendation is now seen as restrictive and it is accepted that individual women of different ages and abilities should not all be given the same guidelines. For example, let's take an unfit 40-year-old pregnant woman. If she exercised at 140 bpm she would be working too hard. On the other hand, a pregnant 22-year-old fitness enthusiast exercising at 140 bpm would feel she was working reasonably hard but not excessively.

It is now recommended that you should work no harder than 70–75 per cent of your maximum heart rate when pregnant. However, during your pregnancy your heart rate is higher than usual, so this is not a particularly reliable method of measuring intensity. While it is not recommended that you rely on heart rate monitoring alone during pregnancy, when used alongside *rate of perceived exertion* (see below) it can provide accurate results. Another easy method is the *talk test* (also described below). A combination of all three methods offers the best way to get an accurate overall picture.

Talk test

This method of measuring your exercise intensity is simply what it says: while doing cardiovascular exercise you should be able to maintain a normal conversation. In your warm-up sections you should feel able to sing – although if your voice is anything like mine, people may prefer it if you don't! During the main part of your exercise activity you should feel able to talk comfortably. If you are taking a power walk with a friend or colleague you should be able to chat to each other quite easily all the way – a good chance to catch up on any gossip. If you feel too out of breath to talk then slow down – you are working too hard.

Rate of perceived exertion (RPE)

Imagine your level of activity on a scale of 1 to 10, where 0 indicates that you are not doing any kind of physical activity at all and 10 indicates that you are working as hard as you possibly can at a level that you would be unable to sustain for more than a few minutes.

Although it may take you a while to get the hang of this method, it is a very useful tool for measuring how hard you feel you are working every time you do an activity. And it's not a method that should be reserved for when you are working out – next time you are cleaning the kitchen or popping to the local shop for a paper, think about how you would rate yourself on the scale shown in Table 9.1.

Each of you will have different starting levels of fitness, and just as each of you will have a different pregnancy, each one of you will feel different when exercising. When exercising during pregnancy you should avoid exercise at any level above 7. If you are new to cardiovascular exercise start with a maximum of 5 then gradually build up to 6. If you are already fairly fit and used to doing cardiovascular exercise you should aim to work at level 7, and work for longer if necessary rather than harder.

Post-workout fatigue

Fatigue is a common complaint during pregnancy, and you can't get away from the fact that at various times during your pregnancy you will feel tired. If you feel too tired to do your normal workout try a 20-minute walk instead. This will help increase your circulation and give you some of those feel-good hormones.

If you are so exhausted the day after your workout that you feel fatigued and unable to go about your normal daily activities then reassess your level of activity and what you are doing. Perhaps you are doing too much for the stage of your pregnancy.

Table 9.1 Exertion rating scale (RPE)

0	No exertion at all (sitting watching TV or reading)
1	Minimal exertion
2	Very light activity
3	Fairly light activity
4	Light activity
5	Somewhat hard but easily maintained activity
6	Quite hard activity, can be maintained but you will feel a little sweaty and breathe a little deeper and quicker
7	Hard
8	Very hard
9	Extremely hard (can only be sustained for short periods of time)
10	Maximum exertion (can't be sustained for more than a few minutes)

Listen to your body

The two case studies on the next page show that one woman's stroll is another woman's fast walk. Using RPE monitoring worked for both Chrissie and Julie – it was easily used and understood. Both women could use this method when exercising alone and as a rough guide to ensure they do not work too hard. Combining this method with a heart rate monitor and the talk test will give you an accurate picture of how hard you are working. Remember, though: if it feels too much for you then it probably is! Stop and rest, and don't push yourself too hard.

Chrissie's case study

Armed with sensible shoes and plenty of water, I took one of my clients, Chrissie, out on a power walk around the hills of Glossop. She was seven and a half months pregnant at the time. Chrissie is an exercise teacher so she does regular exercise, and she already has a three-year-old child.

After five minutes of easy walking on a flat level she said she felt she was at rate of perceived exertion (RPE) level 3, and could carry on at that level for a long time. She felt that the level was so easy that her back would ache before she started to feel out of breath or tired. We upped the pace and after 12 minutes of power walking up a few slight hills she said she felt she was at RPE level 6. Chrissie said she could maintain this for a good while longer but did feel she was breathing a little deeper; also, she had taken off her sweatshirt.

After a further 15 minutes of walking with seven minutes of power walking we hit a steep hill. Within two minutes of walking up the hill Chrissie said she was at RPE level 8. We were only a third of the way up the hill, and I felt that to continue may place too much of a physical demand on her. Walking up steep hills in mid- to late pregnancy is not advisable because it can place unnecessary strain on the pelvis and back, so we decided to make our way down and take the longer way round. It did mean that our total walk time was an extra 5 minutes, and although we maintained a good power-walking pace we never went above RPE level 6. Chrissie was able to talk all the way through and although she was warm she did not feel hot. In total we had a good 45-minute CV workout.

Julie's case study

When Julie became pregnant with her first child aged 40 she was not as fit as she had been. The previous year she was fitter, and had been attending two aerobic or stability ball classes per week. She had given these up due to work commitments. When she found herself pregnant she was so tired that all she could do was work, eat and sleep. Due to the fact that she has decided to have her first baby later in life she was a little afraid of doing anything that might put the baby at risk.

Julie approached me for personal training in her second trimester at 22 weeks of pregnancy. It was a lovely day and Julie had on good footwear so we went for a walk near where I live, on a reasonably flat surface that has an almost unnoticeable incline (the Longdendale Trail). Once we had got out of the car, I asked Julie how she felt; she said RPE level 1 was a good description.

We walked at a normal strolling pace for the first seven minutes. I spent longer on the warm-up with Julie than I did with Chrissie (see Case study 1) due to her lower level of fitness. Julie said that she felt she was working at RPE level 5; we were only strolling so I chose to stop for few minutes while we did a variety of leg stretches, and this allowed Julie to recover.

We then continued to walk at only a slightly faster pace for another five minutes. Julie said she felt she was working at RPE level 6. We stopped and sat down for two minutes and had a drink of water.

We then walked back to the car at a moderate walking pace. I wanted Julie to be able to talk easily to me on our return journey so we gradually reduced the intensity of the walk until she had recovered to RPE level 2. In total we had a low level 24 minute walk with two breaks.

■ 10. Gym work for beginners

There are many reasons why going to the gym can be a good way to exercise. It is a safe environment, and it doesn't matter what the weather is like outside. There should always be people around to advise about correct technique, and it can be a good way to meet other like-minded people. It will also offer you a range of activities to keep you occupied – most gyms have swimming pools and offer specific exercise classes. It is also well worth checking if your local gym has any specific pre-natal classes.

You may be new to the gym or you may already be a fully paid-up regular member. In this chapter you will find a programme for those of you who are just starting out. If you already use gym machines regularly then skip straight to Chapter 11.

Warming up

Whether you are pregnant or not it is always important to warm up. However, when you are pregnant your heart rate and blood pressure will rise at greater speed at the start of your activity than when you were not pregnant, so a well-planned and gradual warm-up is more important than ever.

A warm-up can help prevent injury and can also ensure that your heart rate and blood pressure will rise only slowly and gradually, making exercise safer for you and your baby. A warm-up is designed to prepare the body for the activity to follow by increasing the heart and breathing rates. This ensures that the body gets sufficient oxygen to allow it to work harder and enables it to get rid of excessive by-products (carbon dioxide and heat) quickly.

A warm-up will also do just what it says: it should warm up your muscles and help lubricate your joints. If you spent five minutes warming up before you were pregnant then you need to increase the amount of time you spend on your warm-up but reduce the level of activity and make the gradual increase in intensity slower and smoother.

Cooling down

Cool-down rules in pregnancy are very similar to those for the warm-up. A cool-down is very important following periods of activity and the aim is to gradually reduce the level of intensity. When you are pregnant it will take longer for your heart rate to return to its resting level, so a good cool-down is essential. It will help you gradually reduce your breathing intensity and heart rate, and aid your recovery. It can also serve to alleviate muscle tension and will help prevent blood pooling in the legs. (This is caused by suddenly stopping aerobic activity, which means that the extra blood being pumped around your body to your heart, lungs and working muscles is allowed to, literally, pool in the extremities.)

At any stage of pregnancy you should cool down gradually for at least five minutes; during your second and third trimesters, decrease the intensity slowly and walk for longer to ensure you have fully recovered and brought your heart rate down.

Once you have completed your cool-down you can move on to stretches (see page 137).

A beginner's guide to gym machines

If you are a complete newcomer to the gym, the treadmill and stationary cycle are the best machines to get started on.

Treadmill

Walking on the treadmill is one of the best cardiovascular workouts you can do when you are pregnant. It helps keep your legs and bottom strong (as well as firm), increases circulation and helps to keep your pelvis mobile. Walking can vary from gentle strolling to faster power walking, so it is adaptable to all fitness levels.

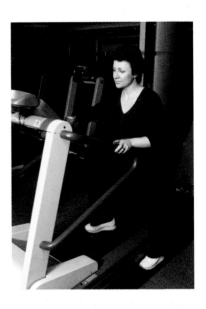

Treadmill tips

- Always step on to the treadmill from the side and make sure it is not moving as you get on it.
- Get a gym instructor to show you how to get on and off safely and how to switch on the machine at its lowest level.
- Use an electric treadmill rather than a manual one, as the pace is more constant.

- Gradually increase the speed of the treadmill until you are walking at a steady pace.
- Always ensure you can talk during your workout.
- Use your arms in a pumping action in time with your legs.
- Make sure you stand tall on the treadmill.
- Avoid gripping the handles or leaning forwards.
- Ensure you take sips of water throughout your workout.
- Breathe normally throughout your workout.
- Ensure you wear good-quality training shoes.
- Wear a well-fitting and supportive sports bra for your workout, which has been fitted by a professional. You may have to buy new ones as your bust size continues to increase.

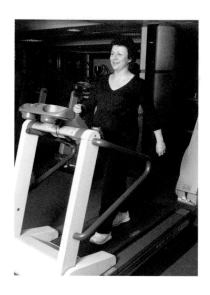

While walking on the treadmill, try to imagine that you are drawing your hip bones closer together (this is just a visualisation exercise – they do not actually move). The resulting abdominal contraction should be minimal and you should feel that you could maintain it throughout your workout. It is a good idea to start practising this early in your pregnancy as long as you have your doctor's permission, are well and have a low-risk pregnancy. If you let your tummy relax this will leave your back unprotected as you walk. This in turn will increase the curve in your lower back and put pressure on your spine and pelvis. It will also strain the abdominals in later pregnancy and possibly increase any gap in the abdominal muscles.

Stationary cycle

The stationary cycle is another good machine to use during your pregnancy. In the third trimester, however, you must take extra care when getting on and off the cycle.

To mount the machine, sit on the cycle seat side on and bring one leg over the middle bar to reach the pedals. Try to avoid lifting the leg very high as this may strain your pelvis. You may find that as your tummy grows your knees start to hit your bump; however, if you increase the height of the seat your legs will have to straighten too much and this may cause strain. So, once you reach this stage, you will have to find an alternative way of getting your cardiovascular workout.

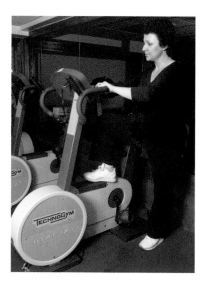

Stationary cycle tips

- Get a gym instructor to show you how to set up the machine and ask him/her to set the pedals up for you at the correct height.
- Avoid wearing G-string underwear when cycling.
- Draw your hip bones closer together, keep your spine long and draw your shoulders down and away from your ears. Avoid over-gripping the bars and leaning forwards.
- Every few minutes, check your posture and do five shoulder squeezes.
- Take regular sips of water.
- If possible, use a gel seat cover to help make the ride a little more comfortable!

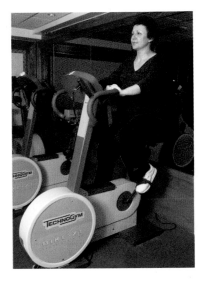

Gym programme for beginners

- Remember to get the go-ahead from your medical care team before you start any exercise programme.
- Start very gradually and build up slowly.
- Always make sure you warm up and cool down properly.
- Start with one to two workouts per week, and aim to increase this to three to five workouts per week when you feel able.
- Start working at RPE level 4, and build up to RPE level 5 at the hardest part of your workout.
- Ensure that you can hold a conversation while exercising.

Table 10.1 on pages 62–3 shows an example beginner programme using gym machines. You can adapt it to meet your own needs, but only move on to the next week's programme once you feel comfortable with the current level. Otherwise simply repeat the week's programme you are already working on – there is no pressure!

Table 10.1 Beginner's six-week starter programme

WEEK	Mon	Tues	Weds	Thurs	Fri	Sat	Sun
1	**Warm-up** On the treadmill, walk at a slow pace with small arm action for 2 mins; work on your posture and breathing **Workout** Gradually increase the pace of your walk and arm action to RPE 3–4 Carry on walking for another 3 mins at RPE 4–5 **Cool-down** Gradually reduce the pace and arm action over 3 mins until you reach RPE 3 Walk for a further 2 mins at a slow pace with limited arm movements at RPE 2	Rest Make sure you start your pelvic floor exercises (see pages 43–4)	Repeat Monday's workout	Rest Start your basic core stability exercises (see pages 35–41)	Rest	Repeat Monday's workout	Try to go for a relaxing afternoon walk, avoiding any steep hills
2	Repeat week 1's Monday workout Increase the maintenance section from 3 to 5 mins if you feel ready	Rest Don't forget your pelvic floor and basic core stability exercises	Repeat Monday's workout	Rest	Rest or try to find a specific pre-natal exercise class for conditioning that is specific to your stage of pregnancy and level of fitness	Repeat Monday's workout	Take a relaxing walk or gentle swim
3	Repeat week 2's Monday workout Increase the maintenance section from 5 to 7 mins if you feel ready Alternate walking at a brisk pace at RPE 5 for 1 min and at a steady but slower pace for 1 min at RPE 3–4	Rest Don't forget your pelvic floor and basic core stability exercises	Repeat Monday's workout	Rest	Rest or attend specific pre-natal exercise class	Repeat Monday's workout	Take a relaxing walk or gentle swim

WEEK	Mon	Tues	Weds	Thurs	Fri	Sat	Sun
4	Repeat week 3's Monday workout. Keep alternating between brisk and slow pace walking.	Rest Don't forget your pelvic floor and basic core stability exercises	Repeat Monday's workout (or swim for the same amount of time) Note that, if you swim, you will be using different muscles, so take your time and build up the intensity only slowly Rest Pelvic floor	and basic core stability exercises	Repeat Monday's workout	Rest	Take a relaxing walk or gentle swim
5	Repeat week 4's Monday workout You can keep the level the same as above if you feel you are working hard enough, however if you feel ready to increase your workout intensity then work at the same RPE but increase the maintenance section to 9 mins	As above	Repeat Monday's workout	As above	Repeat Monday's workout	Rest	As above
6	Repeat week 5's Monday workout Try to build up your maintenance section to 10 mins over the next few weeks; you can work at RPE 6 should you feel ready, otherwise work out at a lower intensity if it feels better for you	Rest Core stability and pelvic floor exercises	Repeat Monday's workout	Rest or do some conditioning exercises	Repeat Monday's workout	Repeat Monday's workout or swim for the same length of time	Rest

Interval training

Interval training on machines is an effective way to work your heart and lungs as well as exercise your legs. It also allows you to work for longer periods as you alternate between harder and easier activity.

Once you feel comfortable with the beginner's programme shown in Table 10.1, you may wish to move on to interval training. Do not start this until you feel comfortable doing 20 minutes of exercise at RPE level 5–6.

Table 10.2 shows an example interval training programme, which can be used if you feel that you want to move on from the beginner's programme outlined above – adapt it to meet your own needs, but only move on to the next week's programme once you feel comfortable with the current level. If you do start to feel over-tired build more rest days into your programme or move down as many levels as you need to.

Table 10.2 Interval training starter programme

WEEK	Mon	Tues	Weds	Thurs	Fri	Sat	Sun
1 and 2	**Warm-up** On the treadmill, walk at a steady pace for 4–7 mins at RPE 3–5 until you feel warm and are breathing a little faster. **Workout** Walk at a slightly faster pace for a further 3–5 mins at RPE 4–6; take the treadmill up to the first incline and walk at a slower pace for 1 min at RPE 4–6. Repeat the above pattern of 3 mins' fast walking on the flat and 1 min slow walking on the incline for 12 mins if you are already used to working for this length of time. **Cool-down** Ensure that there is no incline on the treadmill and gradually reduce the intensity of your walk for 5 mins until you feel recovered; you should be breathing fairly normally and working at around RPE 2.	Rest or take part in a different conditioning activity with which you are already familiar	Repeat Monday's workout	Rest or take part in a different conditioning activity with which you are already familiar. Swimming is a good alternative to walking; it will also take the pressure off your joints.	Complete rest day – light stretching only	Repeat Monday's workout	Complete rest day – light stretching or relaxing outdoor walking only

WEEK	Mon	Tues	Weds	Thurs	Fri	Sat	Sun
3 and 4	Repeat week 1 and 2's Monday workout and add a further 4 mins to your programme. Do 3 mins walking on the flat or jogging (depending on your fitness level) and 1 min on either the first or second incline with a reduction in the intensity of your walk or jog.	Repeat week 1 and 2's Tuesday workout	Repeat Monday's workout	Repeat week 1 and 2's Thursday workout	Repeat week 1 and 2's Friday workout	Repeat Monday's workout	Repeat week 1 and 2's Sunday workout
5 and 6	Repeat week 3 and 4's Monday workout, or if you feel ready you can do the following: • take the incline up to level 2 or 3 • walk/jog on the flat for 2 mins, reduce the intensity but incline the treadmill for 2 mins.	Repeat week 1 and 2's Tuesday workout	Repeat Monday's workout	Repeat week 1 and 2's Thursday workout	Repeat week 1 and 2's Friday workout	Repeat Monday's workout	Repeat week 1 and 2's Sunday workout
7 and 8	Repeat week 5 and 6's Monday workout, or if you feel ready you can do the following: • walk/jog on the flat for 2 mins, reduce the intensity but incline the treadmill for 2 mins • maintain the intensity but add a further 4 mins to your programme • total time in the maintenance programme should not exceed 20 mins unless you were already used to working for longer than this before you were pregnant.	Repeat week 1 and 2's Tuesday workout	Repeat Monday's workout	Repeat week 1 and 2's Thursday workout	Repeat week 1 and 2's Friday workout	Repeat Monday's workout	Repeat week 1 and 2's Sunday workout

Note: the above programme is only a guide, and as your pregnancy progresses you can still use it but you will need to reduce the intensity of your workouts. Even though you may not feel that you are putting in the same effort, you will still be working as hard and reaching the same level of RPE.

Other gym machines

Recumbent cycle

The recumbent cycle is a stationary cycle that has a leaning seat rather than an upright one. Many people recommend the use of this machine over an upright cycle in pregnancy but, personally, I think you should try both as many women find the recumbent cycle uncomfortable on their back. It really is an individual thing. You can of course do a certain number of minutes on the recumbent cycle then switch to the upright cycle to vary the position of your back during your workout.

The seat on a recumbent cycle can be altered to suit your leg length. Again, ask a gym instructor to do this for you.

As with the stationary cycle you may find that towards the end of your pregnancy your knees start to knock into your bump, so you will probably need to find an alternative.

The time spent and intensity level achieved on the recumbent cycle should be the same as that recommended above for the upright cycle.

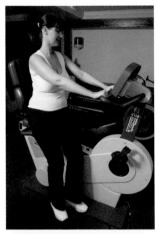

Recumbent cycle tips

- Ensure that you sit upright, draw your shoulders down and away from your ears and think about drawing your hip bones closer together throughout your workout. It is worth mentioning that if you did not cycle outdoors before you became pregnant you should not start to do so now. An indoor stationary cycle is much better for you during pregnancy if you are new to this type of activity.

- Sit on the cycle and think about your technique. Is the leg level and seat level appropriate for you? Feel as if you are drawing your hip bones closer together to slightly contract your abdominals during your workout. Hold on to the handlebars, but avoid over-gripping them, and maintain good alignment of the spine.

- To warm up, cycle slowly for one minute at a low level of resistance.

- Increase your speed for a further minute.

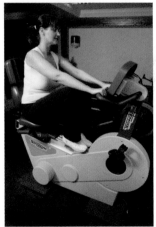

- Increase the resistance of the cycle to the next level for a further two minutes.

- Increase your speed at this level for another two minutes. You should be working at an RPE of 4–5 by the end of your warm-up.

- Maintain this level for five minutes, if you feel that your RPE is getting too high then reduce the resistance level. Gradually increase the time by two minutes each week, until you can do 20 minutes.

- To cool down, gradually reduce your speed and the resistance level on the cycle for approximately five minutes, or until you feel you have fully recovered.

- Once you can maintain 20 minutes you can start to interval train during the main part of your warm-up. You can increase the resistance on the cycle so that you have to work a little harder to push the pedals. Do this for one to two minutes. Then reduce the level of resistance and pedal faster for two to three minutes. Repeat this interval a number of times.

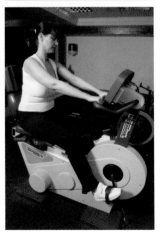

- Don't forget your warm-up and cool-down.

Once you have built up your time to, say, 20 minutes, you could alternate the machines you use to vary the position of your back and work a variety of muscles. I would suggest that, as a beginner, you start to exercise not only with your doctor or midwife's permission but also with the guidance of a qualified gym instructor (who, ideally, is also qualified to teach pre- and post-natal exercise). Refer to the 'Useful addresses and websites' section at the end of the book for helpful contact details.

Rowing machines

A rowing machine is much harder to use in terms of technique. It also uses the arms and legs together so you would be advised to build up to using this machine and initially use a cycle or treadmill for your warm-up. The machine you use should be in good working order, and the rowing action should be fluid and smooth.

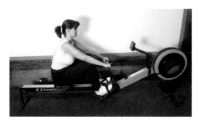

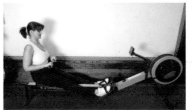

As you really need to be taught to use a rower correctly I would suggest you only start to row under the guidance of a qualified gym instructor. He or she will need to pay particular attention to the position of your back, your arm technique and wrist positioning – even more so now you are pregnant!

Rowing machine tips
- Warm up for between four and six minutes.
- Row at a low resistance and with a steady pace so that you feel you are working at RPE level 4–5. As you become fitter you can build this up to RPE level 6.
- Aim for five minutes initially, then add two minutes to your workout each week until you can row for 20 minutes. If this is too much for your back or you feel it is making you work too hard, stay at, say, 10 minutes' rowing then switch to another machine.
- Cool down gradually for five minutes or until you feel you have fully recovered. If you are cooling down on the rower, spend the last few minutes at the end of your cool-down just using your legs.

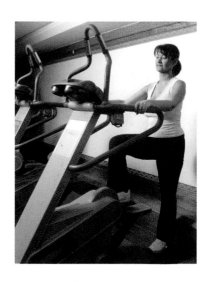

Steppers

Due to the action of the legs required when using a stepper you need good muscle control and stability in your pelvis to use this machine correctly. I would suggest that you start your fitness programme on the treadmill or a cycle before moving on to the stepper. Once you become fitter you could use the stepper for the main part of your aerobic workout;

warm up and cool down on familiar machines, though, and get a qualified gym instructor to show you how to use the stepper correctly. He or she should look at your pelvis from behind and make sure that you do not drop it from side to side; it should move equally up and down to reduce stress in this area.

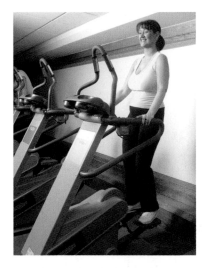

Stepper tips
Follow the guidelines under 'Rowing machine tips', above, once you start to use this machine. The stepper is not ideal for beginners.

Cross-trainers
It is difficult to maintain your balance and control on this type of machine if you have not used one before. The cross-trainer also uses arm and leg actions combined so this may make your heart rate rise quickly; the coordination required is also quite difficult to master if you are not used to it (you can, however, switch off the arm action on some machines). The leg movement involved means that the cross-trainer is a very low-impact machine, and this may make it more suitable for some of you than one or two of the other machines discussed above.

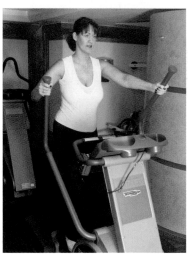

Cross-trainer tips
Start on the treadmill or a cycle to warm up and cool down. (You should also use these machines to help build up your fitness level before starting to work on the cross-trainer.)

As before, get a qualified gym instructor to show you how to use the machine and to help you get on and off it.

Follow the guidelines under 'Rowing machine tips', above, to help plan your workout.

Important note

I would not recommend that you start to use the rowing machine, stepper or cross-trainer if you begin your exercise programme later in your pregnancy. You should stick to the treadmill or cycles instead.

11. Gym work for regular exercisers

The example programmes on pages 74–7 are aimed at those of you who are already regular gym-goers and were using the machines in question before you became pregnant. However, you should still ensure that you get medical consent to exercise while pregnant, and remember to use the rate of perceived exertion (RPE) and talk tests to monitor your exercise intensity.

Table 11.1 Gym machines at a glance

Machine	Stage of pregnancy	Suitable?	Comments
Treadmill	1st trimester 0–12 weeks	Yes – running and walking	As your pregnancy progresses reduce the intensity of your runs to a jog and, if necessary, from a jog to a walk. Pay attention to technique (see the section on treadmill for beginners, pages 59–60).
	2nd trimester 12–28 weeks	Yes – jogging and walking	
	3rd trimester 28–40 weeks	Yes	
Stepper	1st trimester 0–12 weeks	Yes	Stepping is fine in early to mid-pregnancy and you can continue to use the stepper in your third trimester as long as you can maintain pelvic alignment; however the bigger you get the harder this becomes. Use the stepper for only part of your CV work rather than for all of it. In the third trimester I would recommend intervals of no longer than 10 minutes on the stepper. Pay attention to your technique. Avoid stepping if you have sacroiliac pain or sciatica.
	2nd trimester 12–28 weeks	Yes, but with caution	
	3rd trimester 28–40 weeks	Yes, but with caution	

Machine	Stage of pregnancy	Suitable?	Comments
Cross-trainer	1st trimester 0–12 weeks	Yes	The cross-trainer works both the arms and legs at the same time. It can also involve quite a long stride if you are short. Generally, this machine provides a good means of exercise in pregnancy as it is low impact. Use the cross-trainer in your warm-up without the arm action so that you do not raise your heart rate too quickly. Alternatively, you could warm up on a different piece of equipment and use the cross-trainer in the middle of your aerobic component.

Some machines allow you to switch off the arm action; if so, always start without incorporating the arms, gradually add them in and then finish without the arms for a few minutes before you get off the machine. Ensure that you get a qualified gym instructor to teach you how to use this machine if you have not used one previously, and take great care getting on and off. Do start with the legs only if you are new to exercise and work for about five minutes two to three times per week on alternate days. Gradually increase your workout by two minutes every week. Aim to build up to 20 minutes and introduce the arm action in the middle of your workout.

For those of you who are used to using a cross-trainer, carry on! Do make sure you warm up and cool down slowly, though. In the third trimester, use a cross-trainer that allows you to switch off the arm action if you start to find the intensity level too hard. Remember to monitor your RPE and bear in mind that you should feel you can hold a conversation throughout your exercise programme. |
| | 2nd trimester 12–28 weeks | Yes | |
| | 3rd trimester 28–40 weeks | Yes, depending on the machine | |
| **Rowing machine** | 1st trimester 0–12 weeks | Yes | Rowing machines are very suitable for use during pregnancy as they are low impact and work the upper as well as the lower body.

Good technique is essential, however. You will need to get a qualified gym instructor to check on your technique, particularly your back and wrist positioning.

As your pregnancy progresses you may find it more difficult to get up from and down to the floor. You may also find that your growing tummy gets in the way. Once your knees contact your tummy during the rowing action it's time to stop. Avoid compensating for this by taking your knees apart as this will stress the pelvis.

If you have no problems with your rowing technique or knee position then you can continue to row throughout your pregnancy. I realise I am a bit of a nag, but I see so many people rowing with the wrong technique, specifically in the upper body and wrist positioning, that I want you to work hard to maintain the correct |

Machine	Stage of pregnancy	Suitable?	Comments
Rowing machine (continued)			technique. So, to reiterate, get a qualified gym instructor to check your technique at regular intervals.
	2nd trimester 12–28 weeks	Yes/no	
	3rd trimester 28–40 weeks	No	
Stationary cycle (upright)	1st trimester 0–12 weeks	Yes	The stationary (upright) cycle offers an ideal form of exercise in pregnancy as it is low impact. As your pregnancy progresses you will need to take care when getting on and off the cycle in order to reduce the amount of strain placed on the pelvis. You are likely, too, to appreciate the benefits of using a gel seat cover! You must ensure that you focus on good technique throughout. Keep taking rests from leaning forwards, and cycle in an upright sitting position every few minutes to reduce pressure on your lower back. Make sure you do not over-grip the handlebars. If you are unfortunate enough to get any varicose veins in your groin or vagina you may feel that the sitting action is not appropriate. Some of you may find that, as your pregnancy progresses, your tummy gets bigger and your knees start to come into contact with it. Do not adjust the pedal height as this will make the cycling position incorrect for your size, and can stress the pelvis and knee joints. You could try swapping the upright cycle for the recumbent cycle, but you may still meet the same problem. Many of you will not have this problem but some of you are certain to, so change to using the treadmill if necessary.
	2nd trimester 12–28 weeks	Yes	
	3rd trimester 28–40 weeks	Yes	
Recumbent cycle	1st trimester 0–12 weeks	Yes	The recumbent cycle can offer the back more support, but some women find the seat position uncomfortable. You will just have to try it for size. Lots of recumbent cycles allow you to adjust the seat position. It is essential that you get a qualified gym instructor to show you how to do this correctly and to ensure the seat height is right for you. You must also check the seat position in relation to your leg and knee positions. You must be able to lengthen your legs as you cycle, but you do not want to have to lock your knees out straight or feel that you have to move your pelvis in order to

Machine	Stage of pregnancy	Suitable?	Comments
Recumbent cycle (continued)			reach the pedals. Again, one machine will vary from another, and it is advisable to get someone to look at your position on the cycle and check that it is correct for you. You may feel that you can carry on using the recumbent cycle throughout your pregnancy – if it is comfortable and manageable then it is ideal. However, you may find that, as your pregnancy progresses, it becomes uncomfortable to hold a position for long periods of time; you may also feel pinching around the groin area. As mentioned elsewhere in this chapter you may consider it fine to use the recumbent cycle, but it may be best to use it as part of your cross-training programme so that you are not using it for extended periods of time. Eventually, as with the upright cycle, your tummy may get so big that your knees start to come into contact with it. If this happens, you will need to find alternative equipment.
	2nd trimester 12–28 weeks	Yes	
	3rd trimester 28–40 weeks	Yes	
Arm ergometer	1st trimester 0–12 weeks	With caution. See comments opposite.	I have a problem with this machine, which I shall explain as we continue. However, it is only my opinion and I am sure others would successfully justify the use of this piece of equipment. Unless you are confined to a wheelchair or are limited in your lower-limb mobility, then other cardiovascular machines are far more effective at training your heart and lungs, and far more functional (i.e. offer benefits for everyday life). Because this machine focuses on the upper body you have to work quite hard to get a training effect on the heart and lungs. And, because the activity is only in the upper body, you may increase your heart rate quite quickly. Your legs will not be used at all and as a result will not benefit in any way from this type of training. Due to the upper-body action involved, you may also find that use of this machine can increase your blood pressure. As your pregnancy progresses, your tummy will get in the way of you reaching the hand paddles – unless you have very long arms! However, if you are specifically involved in a sport or activity that only uses the upper body, or you are restricted in the use of your legs, then this machine may be of value. If you are disabled in the lower body or confined to a wheelchair, however, then you must seek advice beyond that offered by this book. I am sure you will be able to work with a programme specifically developed for you and I hope you continue to exercise throughout your pregnancy, however you will need to seek additional medical advice and guidance if you wish to do so.
	2nd trimester 12–28 weeks	With caution. See comments opposite.	
	3rd trimester 28–40 weeks	With caution. See comments opposite.	

Machine	Stage of pregnancy	Suitable?	Comments
Air walkers	1st trimester 0–12 weeks	Yes	The air walker is not commonly found in all gyms. It is a machine that does not involve any movement in the knees. The arm and leg action called for is similar to that of skiing. This wide-leg movement from the hip is not good for the natural movement of our bodies and can put stress on the pelvis, therefore limiting its suitability for use during pregnancy. In addition, the arm movement involved when using this machine may mean that the heart rate is elevated too quickly.
	2nd trimester 12–28 weeks	Not after 20 weeks	
	3rd trimester 28–40 weeks	No	
Ski machine	1st trimester 0–12 weeks	Yes	This machine is similarly suited to use during pregnancy as the air walker (see above). However, if you are a competitive skier it may be far safer than skiing outdoors where you could slip or fall. For this reason, and if you are a competitive skier, you could carry on using this machine. However, you must stop if you have any problems with your pelvis, knees or back. Reduce the length of your stride and arm action as your pregnancy progresses.
	2nd trimester 12–28 weeks	Not after 20 weeks	
	3rd trimester 28–40 weeks	No	

Versa climber	1st trimester 0–12 weeks	Yes	This machine involves the use of the arms and the legs in a strong action. You also need to be close to the machine to be able to reach the foot and hand paddles.
			  If you are familiar with this machine you can carry on using it in the first trimester and into the first part of the second. However, I would recommend that you use this in the main body of your cardiovascular workout only, and use an alternative machine to warm up and cool down.
			  The intensity levels required by this machine may mean that it is inappropriate for use from approximately 20 weeks of pregnancy. You will also struggle to reach the foot and hand paddles as your tummy gets bigger!

	2nd trimester 12–28 weeks	Not after 16–20 weeks	
	3rd trimester 28–40 weeks	No	

Guide to working out for experienced exercisers

The following programme is for those of you who were already using gym machines as part of your training programme before you became pregnant. The programme may also be suitable for those of you who ran or hill-climbed outdoors and feel you need an alternative training method now that you are pregnant.

As every woman has a very different experience of exercising when pregnant, it is impossible to give workout programmes with exact times and levels. The guidelines below are based on measuring your rate of perceived exertion (RPE), and this will be different for everyone. To understand how to measure your RPE and other methods for seeing how hard you are working refer back to pages 55–6.

1st trimester **0–12** WEEKS	Provided that yours is a low-risk pregnancy (see page 18 for a definition of this) and you are fit and healthy, you should be able to carry on with your exercise programme as normal. **General guidelines** • Never exercise above RPE 7 (see page 55–6) • Take extra rest days if you feel more tired than normal. • Drink extra water during and after your workouts. • Take care not to get overheated during your workouts. • Avoid working out if you are ill.
1st part of the second trimester **12–20** WEEKS	**General guidelines** • Always monitor your exercise intensity (RPE). • Adjust the level if you are working too hard. • Buy new trainers or a sports bra if necessary. **Warm-up** • Walk at a slow pace on a flat surface for three minutes (RPE 3). Gradually increase the speed of your walk and use your arms more for a further four minutes (RPE 4). • If you are used to running, gradually take it up to a jogging pace for a further five minutes (RPE 5). **Workout** • Jog at an appropriate pace for a further five minutes (RPE 5/6). • Gradually reduce to a walking pace for three minutes (RPE 3). • Switch to a stepper or rowing machine, if you are used to using them, for 8 to 12 minutes (RPE 5/6), slowing towards the end (RPE 3). • Switch to an upright or recumbent cycle for a further 6–12 minutes (RPE 5), then start the cool-down opposite. *Always reduce the intensity of your work before you come off a machine, and only gradually increase the intensity when you move on to a new machine.*

1st part of the second trimester
12–20 WEEKS
(continued)

Cool-down
- Continue with cycling and gradually reduce the intensity until you are hardly moving; this should take between six and eight minutes.
- Ensure you have returned to a low level (RPE 2) before you stop altogether.
- If you prefer, switch to the treadmill to cool down, starting with a power walk and gradually reducing to a slow stroll.

Stretch
- Follow the stretch routine outlined under the heading 'Post-cardiovascular stretches', on page 77.

2nd part of the second trimester
20–28 WEEKS

General guidelines
- Always monitor your exercise intensity (RPE).
- Adjust the level if you are working too hard.
- Don't work above RPE 7.

Warm-up
- Walk at a slow pace on a flat surface for three minutes (RPE 3). Gradually increase the speed of your walk and use your arms more for a further four minutes (RPE 4).
- If you are used to running, gradually take it up to a jogging pace for a further five minutes (RPE 5).
- Alternatively, cycle slowly for a few minutes (RPE 3), then increase the intensity of your cycling for a further five minutes (RPE 6).

Workout
- If you warmed up on the treadmill switch to a cycle; if you warmed up on a cycle switch to the treadmill. Power walk, jog or cycle for 6–10 minutes (RPE 5/6), reducing towards the end (RPE 3).
- Switch machines again to either the rowing machine, stepper, cycle or treadmill. Work on this machine for 5–12 minutes (RPE 5), reducing towards the end (RPE 2).

Cool-down
- Gradually reduce the level of intensity for three to five minutes until you are working at RPE 2.
- If you are rowing or stepping, switch to the treadmill or cycle and follow the instructions above.

Stretch
- Follow the stretch routine outlined under the heading 'Post-cardiovascular stretches', on page 77.

1st part of the third trimester
28–34 WEEKS

General guidelines
- Always monitor your exercise intensity (RPE).
- Adjust the level if you are working too hard.

Warm-up
At this stage of your pregnancy, you will need to increase the duration of your warm-up, but work at a lower level.

- Walk at a slow pace on a flat surface for four minutes (RPE 3). Gradually increase the speed of your walk and use your arms more for a further three minutes (RPE 4).
- Alternatively, cycle slowly for three minutes (RPE 3), then increase the intensity of your cycling for a further five minutes (RPE 6).

1st part of the third trimester
28–34 WEEKS
(continued)

Workout
The level that you worked at previously during your warm-up will now become closer to the level you should work at for your main workout.

- Treadmills, cycles and cross-trainers (without the arm action) are ideal machines to use for this stage of your workout. Some of you may now find the stepper or rowing machine uncomfortable. If they still feel OK, though, continue to use them, but do reduce the intensity.
- Work at RPE level 5–7 for up to 20–30 minutes, depending on how you feel. Maintain a steady level for this period of time or, alternatively, interval train by decreasing and increasing intensity levels.
- You may also wish to use two different machines to make up the main body of your workout. Don't forget to reduce the level of intensity before you get off one machine and gradually increase the intensity as you start on the new machine.

Cool-down
By this stage of your pregnancy it will take longer for your heart rate to recover.

- Gradually reduce the level of intensity at which you are working for five minutes until you are working at RPE 2 and feel fully recovered.

Stretch
- Follow the stretch routine outlined under the heading 'Post-cardiovascular stretches', on page 77.

2nd part of the third trimester
34–40 WEEKS

If you think that your baby's head has become engaged, then you may need to change your workout plans. (See the section headed 'Getting engaged', below, for more information.)

General guidelines
- By now, most of you will find you are working quite hard just walking around and getting through your everyday life, so you will really need to change the intensity of your aerobic training.
- If you still feel fine you can always continue with the workout for the first part of the third trimester, above.
- Ensure you are resting sufficiently, staying well hydrated and eating well, providing yourself with sufficient calories and nutrients.
- If things are getting really hard for you, however, you may wish to move on to a light walking or swimming programme instead.

Warm-up
- On the treadmill, upright or recumbent cycle start with a gentle level of activity for approximately five minutes at RPE level 3.
- Gradually increase the intensity for a further three minutes (RPE level 4).

Workout
You will now find that there is not much difference in the levels of intensity between the end of your warm-up and the main part of your training programme.

- You may need to switch machines to reduce repetitive strain on your joints.
- As before, gradually build up the intensity level on each new machine to a maximum of RPE level 5 or 6 for 10–15 minutes.
- Either work at a constant rate, or interval train by reducing the intensity of your workout to RPE level 3 for two minutes then gradually increasing the intensity to RPE level 6 for one minute. Play around with these times and levels depending on your own particular fitness level.

Cool-down
- Either stay on the machine you are using or change to a different machine.

2nd part of the third trimester

34–40 WEEKS

(continued)

- Reduce the intensity of your work to RPE 4. Maintain this for two minutes, then reduce your RPE to level 3 for a further two minutes. Now work at a very low rate of RPE 2 until you feel you have fully recovered.

Stretch
- Follow the stretch routine outlined under the heading 'Post-cardiovascular stretches', below.

Post-cardiovascular stretches

Do the following stretches, which you will find described in Chapter 17 on the pages indicated:

- calf stretch (page 138)
- hamstring stretch (page 139)
- quad stretch (page 139)
- adductor stretch (page 140)
- abductor stretch (page 140)
- hip flexor stretch (page 141)
- chest stretch (page 142).

You may feel that the above stretches – particularly those for your hip flexors, chest, calves and hamstrings – also help to release tension before you start your workout. If you wish to do any of these stretches before the main body of your workout, then do them halfway through your warm-up so that you are already warm but not working too hard yet. Bear in mind, however, that there is much controversy surrounding stretching during the warm-up; to find out more about the pros and cons, please read Chapter 17, on yoga and flexibility.

Getting engaged

When your baby is moving into position ready for birth, its head will drop down into your pelvic cavity (an occurrence also know as 'lightening'). This generally takes place two to four weeks before delivery during a woman's first pregnancy, but in subsequent pregnancies is more likely to happen when she goes into labour. Once the baby's head does engage you may see a difference in the shape of your tummy – your bump may seem lower and further forwards. You may also feel that you can breathe easily for the first time in months, as the pressure on your diaphragm is reduced. Eating may also become more comfortable.

Unfortunately, the downside of this stage is that you may feel more pressure on your bladder and find it harder to both control and exercise your pelvic floor. You may have to pee more often (hence more sleepless nights). The pelvic area becomes more stressed, both at the front and back of the pelvis, and you may feel discomfort or pain. You may also feel more off-balance than usual, as your centre of gravity changes yet again. In addition, you might develop the pregnancy 'duck waddle' seen in many pregnant women. This is why it is more important to continue to do some core stability work or Pilates exercises at this stage, to help maintain the stability of your pelvis.

You may find that you cannot do any impact activity comfortably. I would suggest you try walking, stationary cycling or swimming instead.

For seasoned exercisers only!

My friend Julie has always been super-fit and continued to exercise through her pregnancies. On her last pregnancy, she was a little overdue. She had been exercising but had been avoiding impact for the past month. In an attempt to get things going, she went for her normal gym workout and had a number of little runs between walking intervals on the treadmill. Bingo! Later that night Julie went into labour.

Note, however, that this is not something I would approve of had Julie not been overdue and very used to exercise.

12. Walking, running and swimming

Walking

Walking in pregnancy is a great form of exercise, and is also a very good activity to start if you are new to exercise. (See the guidelines for treadmill use in the beginner's programme on pages 59–60.)

Walking outside not only exercises your legs and buttocks, but also gives you an opportunity to get some fresh air and see places that you may not otherwise see while sitting in a car, train or bus. Most people can easily fit some extra walking into their daily lives. It will increase your circulation and release feel-good hormones. The only downside is that you may not always be able to walk in extreme weather conditions – walking in icy conditions or on very hot days is not recommended if you are pregnant.

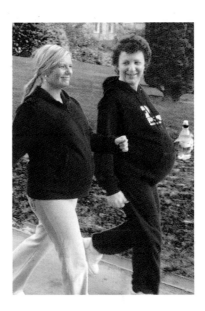

Walking tips

- Try to walk on level, even ground and avoid steep inclines and declines.
- Wear a good and supportive sports bra without wires.
- Invest in good walking shoes or trainers.
- Sip water throughout your walk.
- Move your arms by your sides in a pumping action.
- Keep your elbows close to your ribs and your thumbs pointing upwards.
- Stand tall, keeping your shoulders down and away from your ears.
- Think about drawing your hip bones closer together.
- As you walk, hold your abdominals in – this will help to support your spine and improve your core stability.
- If you live in an area that is hilly, avoid starting your walk on a hill, as this will raise your heart rate too quickly. Finish your walk on a flat surface to ensure that your heart rate lowers.

Basic interval walking programme

- Start with a five-minute warm-up at a moderate walking pace on flat ground at RPE level 3.
- Walk for a further five minutes at slightly harder pace at RPE level 5.
- Alternate between walking three minutes at a moderate rate (RPE 3) and one to three minutes at a faster pace (RPE level 5–6).
- Continue to alternate slow and faster walking for a further 5–30 minutes, depending on your fitness level and stage of pregnancy.
- Always finish your workout with a seven-minute cool-down, gradually decreasing intensity to a steady slow pace.

Interval walking

Interval walking is a good activity for those of you who were already reasonably fit and did a lot of walking before becoming pregnant.

Running

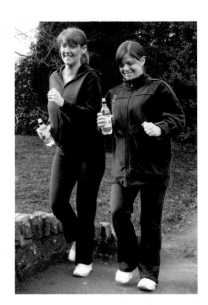

If you were not a regular runner before getting pregnant then now is not the time to start! Walking is a better activity if you are new to exercise. Jogging is preferable to hard running or sprinting after the first trimester.

If you are already a runner then you can continue to run throughout your pregnancy until you feel uncomfortable doing so. Once you feel running is becoming more difficult, start to use a walking programme instead (see that suggested above). Remember that pregnancy is not the time to break records or increase the distance you run. As your pregnancy progresses you need to gradually reduce the intensity of your running. Those of you who were already fit before you became pregnant may find that when you reduce the intensity of your running you may increase the length of time for which you can run.

It is hard to offer a one-size-fits-all running programme, as everybody has different fitness and running experience. However, the guidelines below may help you to plan your running programme when pregnant.

Running guidelines for each trimester

First trimester

For the first 12 weeks of pregnancy you may find that you can warm up the way you did previously. However, it is important that you listen to how your body is feeling and don't put pressure on yourself to work to your pre-pregnancy level. It is quite common in early pregnancy for your heart rate to go up quickly or for you to feel that your heart is racing even when you are not exercising. You may also feel faint or dizzy when standing up or when bending over to do up your running shoes. These are normal symptoms but they should make you sit up and take notice that your cardiovascular system is making adaptations to your pregnancy and consider that you may need to reduce the intensity of your warm-up and make it a little longer and a little slower before you start the main part of your run. On the other hand, you may feel great and may not need to adjust your current warm-up for the first trimester of your pregnancy. Do be aware, though, that even if you feel well, you will overheat far more quickly than normal, and you need to reduce the intensity of your workouts in warmer weather and ensure that you stay well hydrated.

Second trimester
- Start with a walk.
- Gradually increase the speed of your walk for a further three minutes.
- Take time to mobilise (move) the shoulders and neck to loosen up your upper body.
- After a few minutes' walking, you can gradually increase your speed for another couple of minutes (still walking). Aim to walk for about another five minutes before you start to take up a very gentle jogging pace. Stick to this pace for another three to five minutes before running.
- Cool down gradually by walking at a slow pace.

Third trimester
- Start with a slow walk for three minutes.
- Gradually increase the speed of your walk for a further three minutes.
- Take time to mobilise (move) the shoulders and neck to loosen up your upper body.
- Gradually increase the speed of your walk again, for another three minutes.
- Aim to walk for approximately 10 minutes before you start to take up a very gentle jogging pace.
- Cool down gradually by walking at a slow pace.

Swimming
Advantages
Swimming is an ideal form of exercise in pregnancy. It is a good aerobic form of exercise that does not stress the joints. It helps to work the heart and lungs while also conditioning and toning most of the muscles. Swimming also helps improve your circulation and can help alleviate any swelling. The most wonderful thing about any exercise in the water is that the water supports your body weight – suddenly the weight of your baby is gone. You are likely to feel as if a great weight has been taken off your back and shoulders and it literally has! Also any body heat created while you are swimming is dissipated into the water so there is less chance of you overheating. Please note that your heart rate is slower in the water – avoid trying to work as hard with your heart rate or RPE as you would on land.

Running tips
- Always start with a very gradual warm-up.
- From the second trimester, your warm-up should be less intense but longer.
- Always finish your run with a gradual cool-down and wind up at a walking pace.
- From the second trimester, make your cool-down less intense and longer.
- Never exceed RPE level 7 (see pages 55–6).
- Run on level ground – pregnancy is not the time to go cross-country!
- Wear a well-fitting and supportive sports bra with no wires.
- Invest in a good pair of trainers.
- Ensure that you take water with you on your run and sip it throughout.
- You may find that interval training works best for you as your pregnancy progresses.
- If you are running outside make sure somebody knows the route you are taking and the approximate time you expect to get back.
- Take your mobile phone with you.
- Store your water and phone behind you rather than on your abdomen.
- Run with good posture and your abdominals slightly contracted throughout.
- Avoid running up steep hills as this may make the intensity too high.
- Avoid running down steep hills as this can put extra strain on the joints.

Disadvantages

If you have problems with your pelvis, specifically if you have any pain down the front of your pelvis, breaststroke can inflame this area or increase the separation in the pubic symphysis. You can read about this condition (symphysis pubis dysfunction) on pages 163–4. If you do have problems with your pelvis, try swimming without using the breaststroke leg action. Swimming on your back and using floats is a good alternative. Walking in the water is another good option, but you must be careful to avoid any sideways stepping. Treading water with a floatation device may an alternative (see 'Water jogging' opposite).

If you do not have any problems with your pelvis, it should be fine to do breaststroke and many other swimming strokes throughout your pregnancy. When swimming on your front avoid constantly keeping your head out of the water as this will increase the curve in your neck and encourage the lumbar spine to overarch. It may help you to use a snorkel when swimming on your front so that you can breathe without having to keep lifting your head out of the water. Using goggles may help to prevent stinging eyes, but using them is a matter of personal choice.

How long and how hard you swim depends on your pre-pregnancy fitness level, your swimming experience and the stage of pregnancy you are at. If you were a regular swimmer before your pregnancy then you can swim constantly and steadily for a minimum of 20 minutes and build up to 45 minutes (you may be able to do more than this, depending on your level of fitness). Again always tell your medical care team about your exercise plans and ensure they are happy for you to pursue them.

As your pregnancy progresses swimming will become more difficult. As this happens, you can always reduce the speed at which you swim. Another technique I use when taking my heavily pregnant clients into the pool is to alternate swimming with jogging or walking in the pool.

To conclude, swimming will be good for most of you during your pregnancy. Do take on board the advice given above. Remember, too, that the one thing swimming is not is a weight-bearing activity – this means that the bones are not loaded so there is no increase in bone mass, which is essential for preventing osteoporosis. With this in mind, if possible combine swimming with walking or a specific pre-natal fitness or Pilates class to help increase your bone density.

Swimming tips

- Work on your breathing when swimming; it is important you do not hold your breath.
- Do not jump into the water feet first; this may cause trauma to your tummy or force water into the vagina.
- Do not do butterfly stroke after the first trimester as this can over-arch your lower back and stretch your shoulders.
- Do not swim immediately after eating.
- Do not swim alone.
- Avoid diving into the water after 20 weeks of pregnancy unless you are a very experienced and competent diver.
- Start with a gradual warm-up and finish with a gradual cool-down.
- Use a variety of different strokes.
- Use a variety of equipment, such as floats and woggles.
- Alternate various strokes and pieces of equipment.
- Do not swim on your back if you feel dizzy or faint.

Swimming for beginners

My first question is 'Can you swim?' If not, you could look for a specific pre-natal aqua class. If you can swim but haven't done so for some time then make sure you get your GP or medical care team's approval before you start any exercise programme. If you get the all-clear to go ahead then start with a gentle swim for five minutes. Rest by walking width-wise across the pool for a further few minutes then swim again at a relaxed pace for a further five minutes. Gradually increase your swimming time by five minutes per week. Walk in the water whenever you wish and be careful not to work above level 4–5 (RPE). Once your fitness level increases you will find that you have to swim faster in order to reach your target rate of perceived exertion.

Aim to swim at least twice a week and gradually build up to three to five times per week.

Water jogging

Most people discover water jogging as a form of rehabilitation after injury. (My eldest daughter tells me they also do this with racehorses!) You may, for whatever reason, find that your existing cardiovascular training becomes unsuitable for all or some of your pregnancy. If this is the case, water jogging may be just the thing you are looking for. This form of exercise does exactly what it says: you jog in the water. There are two types of water jogging:

1. you work in water up to or above chest height and jog using your legs and arms under the water
2. you jog in deep water wearing a flotation vest; the vest keeps you afloat, and your feet will not touch the floor; you tread water using your arms and legs.

Method 1 requires you to literally run through the water, whereas method 2 allows you to remain more or less on the spot.

If your feet do come into contact with the floor, then use the same running action you would on land – just quite a bit slower! If using method 1, concentrate on pushing off from your toes as you land, driving your leg behind you, this will move you forwards as you bring your front knee up below hip level. Lengthen the leg forwards to come into contact with the ground then push off the toe again as above. Keep your fingers together and your arms in the water to increase the

Water jogging tips

- First, get your GP or medical care team's permission to proceed.
- Start with a five- to ten-minute session of water jogging if you are pregnant and not used to the exercise.
- As you are working in the water you should not feel yourself getting as hot as when exercising on land.
- Work at RPE level 3–5, depending on your fitness level and stage of pregnancy.
- Avoid overcrowded pools, as you do not want to risk being kicked in the abdominal area.

Amanda's case study

The example that follows is one that I used with Amanda when she reached 35 weeks of pregnancy. Amanda was a regular exerciser who worked out in the gym twice a week and swam once a week for 30 minutes in her lunch break. As she approached the end of her pregnancy she felt very uncomfortable in the gym. She found getting on and off the machines very difficult and enjoyed the sensation of support that she felt in the water. Amanda asked me to train her in the water so she could maintain her fitness levels.

Amanda got into the pool from the steps and walked five widths at the shallowest end of the pool with the water at waist height. She kept her elbows in by her ribs and pumped her arms as she walked. Throughout her walking I encouraged Amanda to keep her abdominals pulled in slightly so that the baby was drawn a little closer to her back; this also helped her to lengthen her spine. She kept her shoulders down and away from her ears, and her neck long.

Amanda then moved into deeper water so that her tummy was completely covered and the water was at chest level. She then walked and jogged for a further four widths. We then did a series of mobility moves in the pool and a couple of stretches to release any tight muscles before she swam.

She then alternated one-length breaststroke and one length on her back, holding a float against her chest and using a kicking-leg action. She repeated this for a total of four lengths. We then stopped swimming and returned to width-walking and jogging using the arms and legs. The swimming and width-walking was then repeated. We then moved on to a 10-minute session of water exercises using water weights and woggles.

Amanda finished with a gentle swim using whatever stroke she felt comfortable with for a further five minutes. She reduced the intensity gradually and then finished with some pool stretches and pelvic floor work. The whole workout took a total of 45 minutes. Amanda was able to continue with similar workouts three times a week until her baby boy was born. Funnily enough, he too loves his regular visits to the swimming baths!

resistance; use your upper body in an opposite-arm-to-leg action, scooping up water and pushing it behind you.

Mix and match

You can always use water jogging as an alternative to continuous swimming. Alternate between swimming two lengths and jogging two widths or whatever combination is best for your fitness level and stage of pregnancy. You can also interval train by water jogging at a high level (moving quickly, with the legs just below hip level for a few minutes) then at a lower level of speed (with the legs kept lower) for your recovery phase.

Water jogging can be very useful but it does tend to be a bit on the boring side. Try to meet up with other mums-to-be so that you can chat as you jog or time each other's interval training.

Water stretches

After your swim or water jog, you can do stretches in the water too, using the walls of the pool for support. If you prefer, you can of course do your stretches by the side of the pool or in the changing room, but take care not to slip.

Important note

Do not use pools or do any sort of water exercise if your waters have broken, as you are at risk of infection.

13. Exercise classes

Exercise classes are a great way to keep fit. They keep you motivated, keep you moving and can be a good way to meet other people. Just because you are pregnant doesn't necessarily mean that you can no longer take part in a regular class or think about starting a new one.

This chapter looks at the different types of classes available, and whether they are suitable during pregnancy. Remember to always let your instructor know that you are pregnant before starting an exercise class; they may be able to offer suggestions and modifications that make the classes more effective for you.

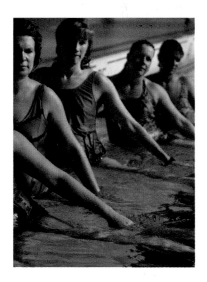

'Normal' aqua classes

If you had been taking part in regular aqua aerobic classes before you became pregnant then they are a great form of exercise for you to continue. You will need to inform your teacher that you are pregnant, though. As long as yours is a low-risk pregnancy you should be able to carry on as normal for your first trimester.

Even into your third trimester you should be able to carry on with your aqua class as the water supports your body weight and there is less stress on your joints than is the case with out-of-water exercise. The weight of the baby is also supported in the water making it easier for you to keep your spine in alignment, and maybe giving you a welcome sensation of lightness!

If possible combine swimming with walking or a specific pre-natal fitness or Pilates class to help increase your bone density. Exercises done in the pool don't bone-load as well as other forms of exercise and some of your stabilising muscles may not have to work as hard as they do on land.

Aqua class considerations

During pregnancy, you will need to make adaptations to normal aqua aerobic exercises; your teacher should be able to help you with this.

Lots of aqua classes involve sideways moves. For example, you may do a series of wide squats from one side of the pool to the other. While wide squats in the water do not place too much pressure on the front of the pelvis in themselves, greater pressure is exerted when you travel as you squat. Some of you may use water-based movements if exercise on land becomes uncomfortable. However, if you have any problems with the front of your pelvis the travelling sideways moves in the pool are more stressful than on land as you have to push against the resistance of the water as you move your legs out and bring them back in again. (On land you would only be working against gravity.)

This specific exercise may require adaptation. You can do this by turning and walking forwards as the group travels sideways, and then turn and walk forwards again as the group moves back to the other side.

Aqua natal classes

Should you be lucky enough to find an aqua natal exercise class near you then this is an ideal form of exercise for those of you who are pregnant and deconditioned. For those of you who are already fit you may find that towards the end of your pregnancy you start to find your normal exercise programme uncomfortable; if this happens, then an aqua natal class would be a good alternative.

Look for a class where the teacher chats to you on the first occasion you join the class. You may find that a midwife either teaches the class or attends the session (see the section below, though).

Two of my very good friends, Christine North and Dawn McClane, are experts in the field of exercise and pregnancy and run a company called Aqua Fusion. They train midwives to teach aqua classes, both pre- and post-natal, and offer courses all round the UK and abroad. Dawn says that aqua natal aerobic classes are specifically designed with the pregnant woman in mind: the water supports the baby *and* your joints so it is a great form of exercise for mums-to-be.

Please refer back to the box entitled 'Considerations for aqua aerobics' as the points made therein also apply to aqua natal classes.

Aqua natal classes and the midwife

Midwives are, obviously, professionally qualified and experts in their field, but this does not mean that they are necessarily also experts in fitness and pregnancy – they are busy enough already! However, midwives who have done courses such as those offered by Aqua Fusion (see above) will be well trained and qualified in both fields. You may wish to refer to the 'Useful addresses and websites' section at the end of this book to find out more, or contact your local swimming pool (many local authorities offer aqua natal exercise classes).

Water polo and high board diving

Both these forms of exercise are not recommended after your 12th week of pregnancy, and I would only suggest you do them before that if you are very used to them! Neither of these types of exercise should be started once you are pregnant. In any case, I expect that if you've just found out you're pregnant one of the last things on your mind is becoming a high board diver!

Aerobics classes

Aerobics can be a great way to exercise because the classes are carefully structured, allowing you time for a warm-up and cool-down. Your teacher should be able to offer you low-impact alternatives to some of the exercises. Attending a class gives you a specific time and place for you to exercise, and it can also be a time to get together with friends and meet new people. See table 13.1 overleaf.

If you are pregnant and new to exercise...

...now is not the right time to start any type of boxing aerobics, kick aerobics, circuit training, high-impact aerobics or complex high-level aerobics. Indeed, you should exercise particular caution before starting *any* class unless it is specifically designed for pregnant women. Most standard classes are an hour long and this is a long time if you are unfit. As long as you are generally active in your everyday life, though, have the OK from your GP and yours is a low-risk pregnancy then you could start a complete beginners' aerobic and conditioning class.

If possible, look for a specific pre-natal pregnancy class or a personal trainer who is qualified in this area. I would also *highly recommend* that you follow the walking programme described in this book on page 79 until you can walk at a steady pace for 30 minutes before you start any beginners' aerobic class.

If you are new to exercise and more than 16 weeks pregnant I would suggest that now is not the time to start any mainstream exercise class. Instead, you should look for something specifically aimed at pregnant women or follow the guidelines for beginners given in this book (Chapters 9 and 10).

Table 13.1 Guidelines on taking part in aerobic exercise in each trimester

Stage of pregnancy	General advice
1st trimester **0–12** WEEKS	You can continue to take part in a variety of aerobic classes as normal during your first trimester as long as you are already used to these classes, have your GP's consent and yours is a low-risk pregnancy. Make sure you have read the previous chapters in this book. If you suffer from symptoms common in early pregnancy, such as initial vascular under-fill (see page 12), you may find that you have to tone down the activities during your class – not that it will do you or your baby any harm but because you may feel like your body is on a go-slow!
1st stage of 2nd trimester **12–20** WEEKS	At this stage of your pregnancy you should start to omit propulsion moves and plyometric moves (intense jumping actions). Use the low-impact alternatives described below. Start to monitor your RPE more – you should always feel that you could talk throughout your class. Don't work at RPE level 7 or above.
2nd stage of 2nd trimester **20–28** WEEKS	At this stage of your pregnancy you should have omitted most impact activities and any turns or twists and replaced them with marching out or jogging on the spot.
3rd trimester **30–40** WEEKS	At this stage of your pregnancy you will all vary in the type of activity you feel comfortable with – some of you will still feel fine when jogging, while others may feel that they want to take out impact moves altogether. You must monitor the intensity of your workouts carefully – feel free to march at the back of the room and drink water for a few minutes if the class gets too hard or the rest of the group are doing more complex movements. Your instructor should feel confident for you to stay in the class and should offer you alternatives throughout the class. However, if they don't feel comfortable about this then do respect their position and look for a more appropriate class.

Some general guidelines for those new to aerobics classes

- Find a specific aerobics class for pregnancy, or a beginner's aerobic class.
- If you have any signs of labour stop immediately! Walk or march on the spot until you recover, then seek medical advice straight away.
- Stop if you have any pain or bleeding. Again, walk or march on the spot until you recover, then seek medical advice straight away.
- Avoid high-impact moves.
- Sip water throughout.
- Feel free to slow down or stop at any time if you are not feeling up to it.
- Avoid stopping suddenly unless you feel unwell.
- Monitor the intensity of your workout (use the methods listed on pages 55–6).
- Ensure you feel your baby move at least twice within 30 minutes of stopping the activity.
- Build up the time you spend exercising slowly, limit aerobic work to a maximum of 45 minutes and do not work above RPE level 6 (see pages 55–6).
- Avoid any twists or turns and/or complex choreography.
- Avoid overusing step-touch movements for long periods as these can stress the pelvis.
- Avoid exercising in hot, humid conditions.
- You may have to further adapt the exercises given in your class or move to a specialist pre-natal class if you feel uncomfortable.

Indoor cycling

Over the past decade or so indoor cycling (also referred to as spinning or, sometimes, studio cycling) has become a popular and very effective method of cardiovascular training. Most of the classes I have ever attended or watched have been real killers! However, this doesn't have to be the case – the great thing about indoor cycling is that you can alter the settings (resistance level) on your bike to work as hard as you wish (or just take it easy).

Indoor cycling is not an ideal form of exercise for those of you who are pregnant and deconditioned. If yours is a low-risk pregnancy, though, you may be lucky enough to find a specific class for pregnant women or an absolute beginners' class. Do go and watch the class before you attend and

Spotting a good teacher

- Does the teacher chat to new people and ask whether anyone is injured, pregnant, and so on?
- Does the teacher observe class members and correct them if necessary, or do they simply shout out instructions without teaching you anything about the exercise, how to do it properly and what it is aiming to achieve?
- Does the teacher offer harder and easier options?
- Is the choreography fairly simple?

Note that you may also find that a teacher is reluctant to take you into their class if they have never taught you before and you are pregnant. Please respect their decision as they may not feel experienced enough to deal with your specific condition and requirements.

Table 13.2 Guidelines on taking part in indoor cycling in each trimester

Stage of pregnancy	General advice
1st trimester **0–12** WEEKS **1st stage of 2nd trimester** **12–20** WEEKS **2nd stage of 2nd trimester** **20–28** WEEKS	• Make sure that you don't get overheated in class • Drink plenty of water • Use a gel seat cover • Avoid lifting up out of the saddle for long periods • As your pregnancy gets beyond 20 weeks, avoid cycling out of the saddle as this can take your heart rate too high and put pressure on your pelvis, unless you have the best technique in the world • Avoid working anaerobically (flat out at RPE 9 or 10) at any stage of your pregnancy • Alter the resistance on your bike so you never feel really out of breath • Avoid more than an hour's workout on the cycle • Avoid cycling on consecutive days • Stop classes if you get haemorrhoids • Stop classes if you get recurrent thrush or cystitis • Adjust the resistance on your bike so you can 'coast' when the group is working flat out • Regularly straighten out your back and avoid leaning forwards over the handlebars for long periods • Use regular rest periods on your bike, where your legs still move, but only slowly and at a low resistance • Do upper-back and postural exercises during a rest phase or while 'coasting' on the bike • Ensure you balance the class by doing core stability or Pilates classes on alternate days, as cycling is not great for your posture • Although heart rate monitoring is not as reliable in pregnancy I would suggest using a monitor in conjunction with RPE and the talk test (see page xx)
3rd trimester **28–40** WEEKS	The following considerations are additional to those listed above. • You may now feel that the seat position and your expanding tummy do not work well together • Avoid indoor cycling if you feel it restricts the abdominal area • Do not alter your seat height beyond what is appropriate for your leg length • As you get bigger, you may wish to use a bike towards the back of the class; this will make you feel less self-conscious if you need to take things easier through the more intensive parts of the workout; it will also allow you to get in and out of the class more easily, without squeezing between tightly packed bikes • Do let the instructor know where you are • When you feel the time is right for you, move on to a different form of cardiovascular training such as using the treadmill, recumbent cycle or cross-trainer • Always start any new equipment with good instruction, and exercise caution at all times

Table 13.3 Guidelines on taking part in circuit training in each trimester

Stage of pregnancy	General advice
1st trimester **0–12** WEEKS	• If you are already circuit training you can carry on. However, you may find that an aerobics class has a more regular sustained level of intensity and is easier for you to control.
1st stage of 2nd trimester **12–20** WEEKS	• If you are very fit you can continue to circuit train, however you will need to discuss this with your instructor • Avoid any type of activity that may cause you to fall • Avoid activity where you may come into forceful physical contact with another participant (e.g. sprinting up and down/shuttle runs) • Avoid activity that is anaerobic in nature (very hard, and that can only be sustained for a short time) • Avoid jumping and propulsion-type moves • Avoid exercises done in a prone position (lying on your tummy) • Avoid exercises that directly work the abdominals, such as sit-ups
2nd stage of 2nd trimester **20–28** WEEKS	At this stage of your pregnancy you will need to make massive adaptations to your circuit training class. If both you and your instructor are happy to do this and you feel that the class is still appropriate for you, then you can continue to circuit train. However, you may find that you need to change the type of class you attend – for example, move to a body-conditioning or aerobics class. Many circuit training classes are very busy with a lot going on, and while your own exercises can be adapted, other people may still be running around everywhere and may run into you. Please bear this in mind – along with the following points – when deciding whether to continue with your circuit class. • Avoid any type of activity that may cause you to fall • Avoid activity where you may come into forceful physical contact with another participant (e.g. sprinting up and down/shuttle runs) • Avoid activity that is anaerobic in nature (very hard, and that can only be sustained for a short time) • Avoid jumping and propulsion-type moves • Avoid exercises done in a prone position (lying on your tummy) • Avoid quick changes of position • Avoid having to get up from and down to the floor at speed • Avoid exercises that directly work the abdominals, such as sit-ups • Avoid deep or power squats (normal squats are OK) • Avoid moving lunges or propulsion lunges (lunges on the spot, known as split lunges, are OK)
3rd trimester **28–40** WEEKS	Most of you will now be finding the pace of most circuit training classes too fast and it will be difficult for you to control the intensity of your workout. However, not all circuit classes are advanced in nature and many may not involve high-intensity or difficult activities. If this is the case then carry on. Please re-read all the concerns above, however, and monitor the intensity of your workout throughout. Do ensure that your instructor knows what stage of pregnancy you are at and that he or she is happy for you to remain in the class.

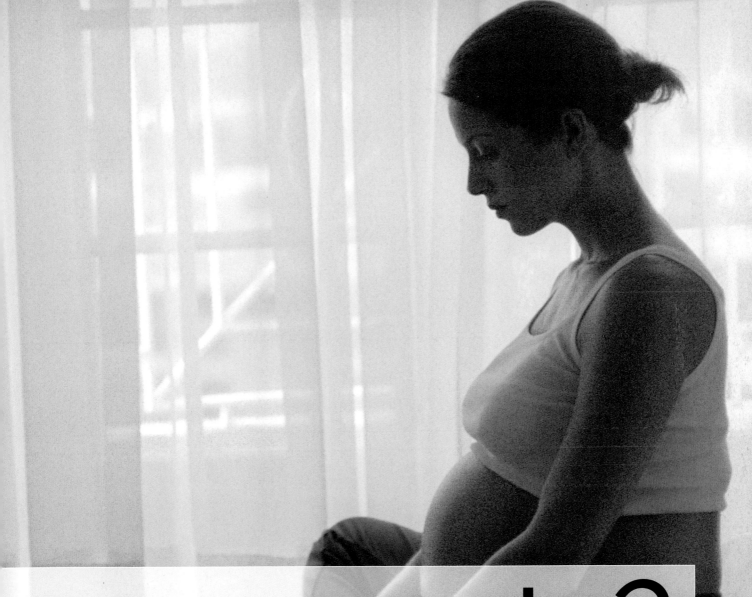

part 3

Resistance training and body conditioning during pregnancy

14. Why resistance train?

Resistance training (using weights or bands to work on specific muscles – see the diagrams below and accompanying box) during pregnancy can have many benefits. It will help to keep your muscles strong enough to support your growing weight comfortably, aid the maintenance of good muscle tone, keep your self-confidence high as your tummy expands and allow you to regain your figure more quickly afterwards.

If you did weight training before becoming pregnant, you may want to continue with it. That's fine, as long as you are aware that you may need to adapt or change exercises as necessary.

If you are not familiar with weight training you could start to do some light resistance training in your pregnancy. You must ensure, however, that you get your GP's consent to exercise and a qualified gym instructor or personal trainer to teach you how to use weights in your circumstances, as a pregnant client.

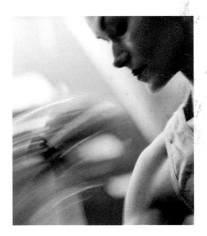

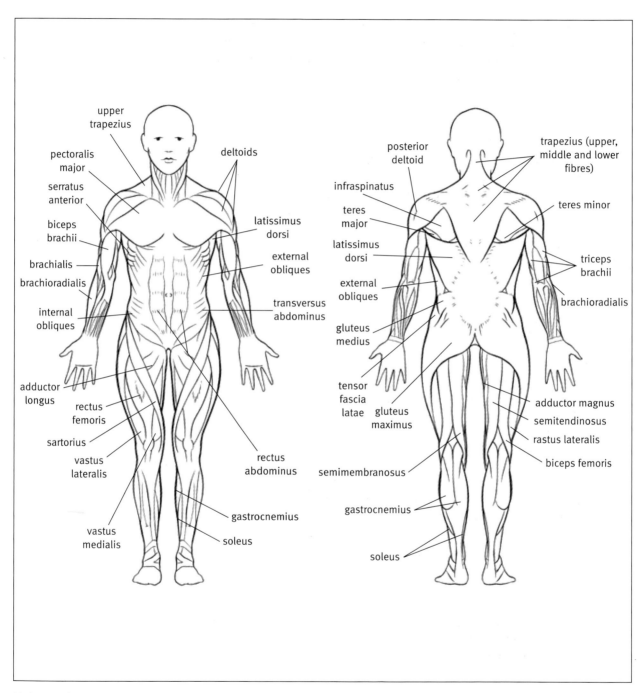

Main muscle groups

I have chosen to include the quite detailed 'musclewoman' diagrams on the page opposite, as throughout many of the following chapters I will be referring to the muscles used. By the end of this book you should be quite the walking anatomy dictionary!

Weight training machines

Weight training machines use static weights; you sit in the machine and use handles or levers to pull or push the weights.

Generally speaking, machine weights do not provide the best way to weight train, as they do not provide the most functional way of training. This is because you often work muscles in isolation and do not have to recruit your core stabilising muscles in order to support yourself – the machines do this for you. However, precisely because some machines make you feel well supported, they may be a good choice for you if you are a complete newcomer to the gym.

Free weights

Free weights are loose weights – either in the form of barbells or dumbbells.

You must always concentrate on maintaining correct posture when weight training. Free weights offer a more effective way to weight train than machine weights because you have to use a variety of muscles to maintain a stable position, good technique and proper alignment.

Body-conditioning programme

Following the body conditioning programme detailed below will help you to maintain your muscle tone and at least some of your strength. Before you start, please read the guidelines below – these apply when doing any kind of resistance training while pregnant.

Breathing

It is important that you do not hold your breath when exercising. Never breathe in and hold your breath as you lift as this can be dangerous during pregnancy. When weight training you should aim to breathe out on the effort during all exercises.

Resistance

As your pregnancy progresses, it is essential that you reduce the load of the weights you are lifting. Table 14.1 offers some guidelines.

Table 14.1 Resistance training advice for each trimester	
Stage of pregnancy	**Resistance training advice**
1st trimester 0–12 WEEKS	During your first trimester you can continue to lift your normal amount of weight. Avoid weight lifting using very heavy weights, though, as this will encourage you to hold your breath while you lift and may increase your blood pressure.
1st stage of 2nd trimester 12–20 WEEKS	In the first half of the second trimester reduce the weights lifted by *at least* 5 per cent.
2nd stage of 2nd trimester 20–28 WEEKS	In the second half of your second trimester reduce this by *at least* a further 5–10 per cent.
3rd trimester 30–40 WEEKS	In the third trimester reduce the weights lifted by *at least* a further 5–10 per cent.

Note: some exercises may put more strain on your back than others, and you may need to reduce your weights further.

Sets and repetitions

Each time you lift a weight it is called a repetition (rep). A number of reps performed together is called a set. After you have performed one set, rest either by stretching, walking around or doing some pelvic floor exercises.

Rest and alternating muscle groups

If you train twice a week, ensure that you do not do your workout on two consecutive days. Go to the gym on, say, Monday and Wednesday. Rest on Tuesday and Friday, and do some cardiovascular training on Thursday and Sunday. For those of you who are training in the gym more than twice a week you should not weight train using the same muscles on consecutive days. For example, if you train your legs, chest

How many?

- New to weight training: one set of your chosen exercises
- Frequent weight trainer: two to three sets of your chosen exercises
- Very experienced weight trainer: two to four sets, depending on the difficulty of the exercise

and triceps on a Monday then work your back, shoulders and biceps on the Tuesday. Rest on the Wednesday and do some cardiovascular exercise on the Thursday. You can also do cardiovascular training on the same days as you weight train. However, as your pregnancy progresses and you get heavier do your leg exercises on days when you do less cardiovascular exercise.

Sets to failure

During pregnancy you should take extra care to use correct technique. Ensure you can manage the weight you use. It is not a good idea to use forced repetitions, where somebody helps you to do the last few reps that you could not do on your own.

It is also better to finish the set feeling you could do a few more repetitions rather than working to failure (when you can't do any more), especially during the third trimester.

Body-conditioning exercises

The exercises on the following pages do not provide step-by-step instructions for using the machines you will find at your local gym. If you are not already familiar with the exercises it is essential that you get a gym instructor or personal trainer to show you the correct technique – machines can vary from gym to gym.

The exercises shown are not a comprehensive list of all resistance exercises that you can do in the gym – there are far too many of them to mention them all here. However, I have selected the exercises that will be most suitable during pregnancy and that, used together, will provide a good and complete workout. I also provide details of how these exercises may need to be adapted as your pregnancy progresses.

Lat pull-down

This machine is suitable for use throughout pregnancy. You may feel that as your pregnancy progresses you are not able to get close enough to the machine due to the roll bar in front of you. Avoid taking the bar behind your neck; bring it down in front of you to the top of your chest instead.

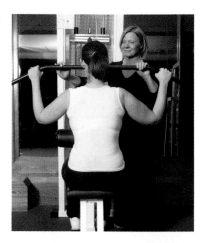

Considerations

- Once your tummy starts to get in the way of the roll bar you may have to adapt the exercise.
- In the third trimester you may also benefit from having a spotter. This is somebody who can bring the bar down for you so you don't have to stretch up to reach it. They can also help take the bar back to its start position when you have finished a set.

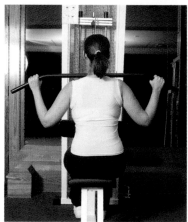

Alternatives

- Standing arm pull-down on machine
- Standing or seated single-arm pulley row

These exercises are a good alternative to the seated row or lat pull-down once these become difficult for you.

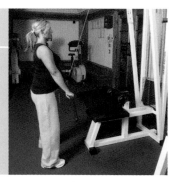

Bent-over row with barbells and dumbbells

This exercise is ideal, as not only does it work important postural muscles, but you also have to work hard on your core stability to maintain good alignment and correct technique.

You may do this exercise standing with a barbell or seated with dumbbells during your first trimester.

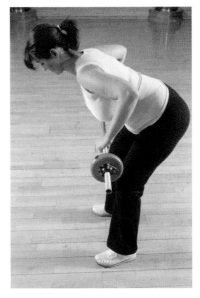

If you were used to doing bent-over rows before you became pregnant you could carry on until approximately 20 weeks of pregnancy then switch to a dumbbell row. If, however, you are new to this exercise you will need to start with a light dumbbell in a supported position.

Considerations

When using a dumbbell you will need to support yourself on a bench or similar (see the picture below). Ensure that you get the bench at the right height to help you maintain correct alignment. You need a strong enough core to maintain a neutral position of the spine (see Chapter 16, page 127) while supporting the weight of your growing baby.

You will need to reduce the weights used in this exercise more than in other exercises to avoid straining your back.

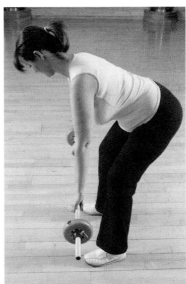

Alternatives

You can also adapt by using the single-arm cable row (ask an instructor to show you).

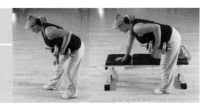

Chest press and incline chest press

From 0–12 weeks, a flat bench press will be fine for you to continue as you did before your pregnancy. You can continue to do an incline bench press throughout your pregnancy but will need to follow the guidelines for the chest press, below.

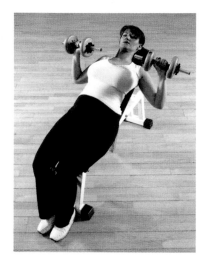

- From 12 weeks switch to using a slightly inclined bench.
- From 20 weeks switch from using a barbell to dumbbells.

Considerations

Incline the bench a little more as necessary, as your pregnancy progresses.

Start to pay attention to how you get on and off the bench.

Once your tummy gets larger you may find getting on to the bench with dumbbells difficult.

Use a spotter. This is somebody who will pass the weights to you and take them from you when you have finished a set.

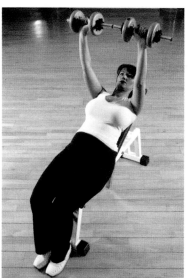

Particularly if you are quite short you may find it difficult for your feet to reach the floor without opening your legs wide. This open-leg position is not good for the pelvis and will cause you to increase the curve in your lower back. This in turn can stress your pelvis, spine and abdominal area. You may find that you can use a step to put your feet on, which will allow you to be able to keep your legs together and make it easier to maintain good spinal alignment.

When you have finished, bring your legs together and turn on to your side, pushing yourself into a seated position, before getting up.

Alternatives - flat flyes and incline flyes

You can continue to do flat flyes for the first trimester, after that you will need to move on to incline flyes. However, the chest press above may leave you feeling more supported after your first 12 weeks of pregnancy. Because your ligaments will be more relaxed, avoid going beyond your normal range of movement. This can place stress on your shoulder joint.

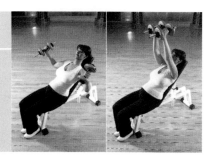

Biceps curl

You can do a standing barbell curl during your first and second trimester.

You can continue to do dumbbell curls throughout your pregnancy.

Considerations

Ensure that you maintain good alignment and keep your spine in neutral throughout the exercise (see Chapter 16, page 127).

Once you find it difficult to maintain good alignment move on to doing a barbell curl in a seated position. To avoid straining your back or abdominal area use alternating biceps curls.

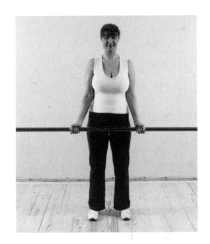

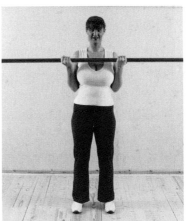

Alternatives

Once the biceps curl using a barbell becomes uncomfortable, you may want to switch to doing dumbell curls – these can be done throughout your pregnancy. Using alternate arms at pictured will help you to maintain good alignment.

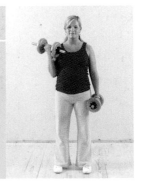

Pulley cross-overs

You need very good core stabilising muscles to do this exercise well after the 12th week of your pregnancy.

Considerations

Work on maintaining good stability and alignment of the spine. You can lean forwards slightly but should not bend forwards. Avoid taking your arms out to the maximum position. You may need to reduce your weight dramatically in this exercise to control the movement and avoid over-stretching the front of the shoulder joint. Aim to keep an even control throughout the movement, and avoid allowing your arms to be pulled back by the machine.

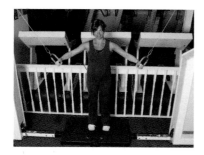
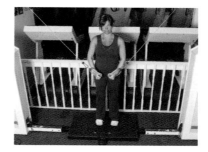

Lateral raise – standing and seated

This exercise is very suitable for use during pregnancy. However, you may find that as you approach the end of your pregnancy you wish to use the exercise in a seated position.

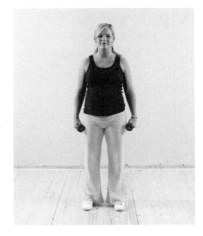

Considerations

Lift the weights to shoulder height only. Work with a slight bend in the elbow to protect your elbow joint. As your pregnancy progresses you must constantly monitor what you are doing in order to ensure that the amount of weight you are using is not encouraging you to adopt poor technique and/or lose correct alignment. You should be able to maintain the position of your body rather than 'throwing' the weights and moving your spine. The lateral raise to the side of the body can be done with both arms as this will help you maintain balance from one side to the other – again, this is likely to mean that you will have to considerably reduce the amount of weight used.

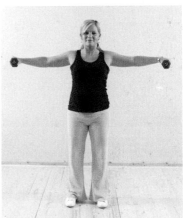

Front raise

As your pregnancy progresses I would suggest you switch to seated front raise. Use exactly the same position as above, but lift the weights out in front of you to shoulder height, using alternate arms.

However, if you feel strong enough to maintain good alignment then continue to do the exercise standing. Do assess, at regular intervals, the amount of weight you use, though, as well as your technique. You should avoid using momentum to lift the weights and should maintain a good neutral spine position throughout (see Chapter 16, page 127).

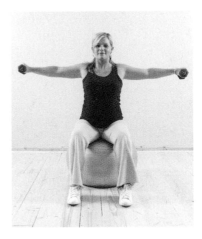

Triceps kick-back

While this exercise can be continued throughout your pregnancy, you will need good core stability to maintain good technique and a neutral spine position (see Chapter 16, page 127). Should you feel stable enough to do this, then use the technique shown below.

Considerations

You may need to switch to triceps press or incline triceps press with a dumbbell if the bent-over position is not comfortable or you struggle to maintain good alignment.

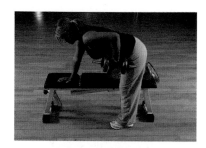

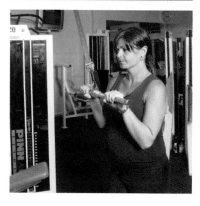

Triceps push-down

This exercise is fine to use during your first trimester and well into the second. You may find, however, that you have to switch to a different exercise once your tummy gets in the way of the bar.

Considerations

You must ensure that you maintain good technique and alignment throughout.

Avoid arching your back during the exercise.

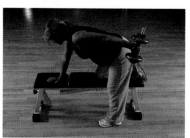

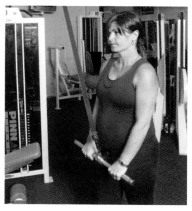

Single-arm triceps press

With care, this exercise can be done throughout your pregnancy, but do take note of the considerations listed below.

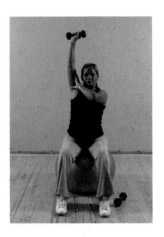

Considerations

After the first trimester, the single-arm triceps press is better than the barbell triceps press.

You can do the triceps press standing or seated. Again, you need to have good stability in standing and need to take care that you do not stand still for long periods of time.

When seated you need to ensure that you maintain neutral alignment (see Chapter 16, page 127) and avoid overarching your back.

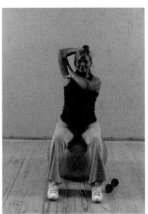

Alternatives

There is also a concern that, after 20 weeks of pregnancy, your blood pressure can be elevated by lifting the weight above your head. At this stage I would suggest you switch to the single arm triceps press using an inclined bench as shown opposite, or the triceps kick-back exercise shown above.

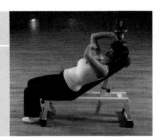

Squats

As long as you do not have problems with your pelvis, spine or knees this exercise is ideal during pregnancy.

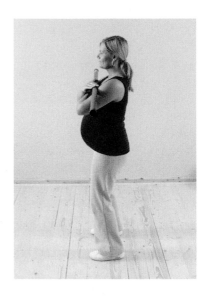

Considerations

It is best to work with the bar in front of you as pictured. You can work with a barbell behind your neck for the first trimester and if you can maintain good alignment and have a good instructor to check your technique you can continue to use the bar until approximately 20 weeks of pregnancy. I am concerned about taking the bar behind the neck, though, as this tends to promote hyperextension of the neck and lower back. This puts stress on the whole of the spine, neck and shoulders. It also makes it harder to preserve the necessary abdominal contraction, which means more stress on the abdominal muscles and less support for the spine.

Switch to using dumbbells when you or your instructor feels you need to – hold one in each hand, with your arms straight down by your sides.

Ensure that you maintain good alignment. This exercise will get progressively harder as you will be lifting more weight as your baby grows. You may feel that you need to reduce the amount of weight used in this exercise more than is the case with some of the others.

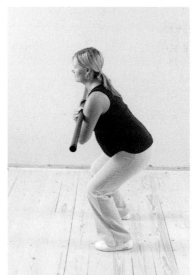

Alternatives

Many women find the wall squats using a stability ball against the wall more comfortable. While this is a good exercise and will help to strengthen the leg muscles I feel it is less of a functional position as you will not actually use this technique in everyday life, when bending down to pick up an object, say. You do not work the buttocks and back extensors as much as you would with the dumbbell squat shown in the picture above.

Lunges

This is tough exercise to do correctly whether you are pregnant or not! However, if you can maintain good technique and have no problems with your pelvis or knees this exercise can be continued throughout your pregnancy with modifications.

Considerations

After your first trimester avoid using a barbell behind your neck and switch to dumbbells instead, or simply use your body weight as you get bigger.

Lunges that involve you stepping forwards and pushing back are a great exercise but it may become difficult for some of you to keep good form and balance as your pregnancy progresses. Switch to using a split lunge, which means you lower yourself down and push up without moving your feet.

You will need to reduce the number of repetitions you do as your pregnancy progresses to avoid overstressing your pelvis and knees. As your baby grows you will find this exercise more difficult as you will have to lift more body weight. You may have to reduce the amount of weight used more than you would do for some other exercises.

If you have any problems with your pelvis then try doing squats (see above) instead of lunges. Both squats and lunges are more functional and use your stabilising muscles more than machines.

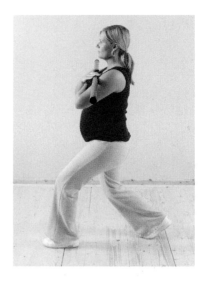

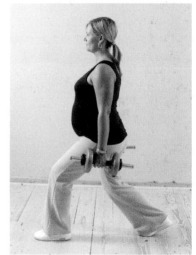

Leg press

There are two types of leg press: the old-fashioned supine leg press, which is done lying on your back, and the more up-to-date leg press, which is done in an incline seated position. It is not appropriate to use the first type of machine after the 12th week of pregnancy. You should be able to use the seated machine until well into your pregnancy, though.

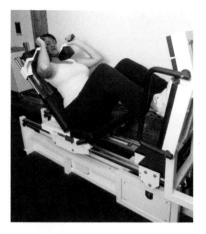

Considerations

There will come a time when you feel you are not able to bring your legs close enough to your body (due to the size of your bump) to do this exercise effectively. The abdominal area will also be crowded and this is something that you need to avoid. Do not compensate for your tummy getting in the way by taking your knees wider as this may stress the symphysis pubis (front of the pelvis).

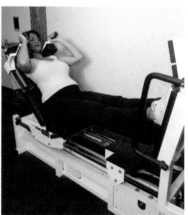

Shoulder press

While this is a very effective exercise for the shoulder muscles it does involve overhead action when lifting the weights above your head, whether you are using free weights or a machine. Free weights are better for your core stability, as the machine supports your spine, meaning that you don't have to do this for yourself.

Considerations

Due to the overhead action involved, this exercise may be inappropriate for you after 12 weeks of pregnancy. If, however, you are very used to this exercise and can maintain good alignment and stability then you could continue until approximately 20 weeks of pregnancy, at which point I suggest you switch to lateral raises (see page 109).

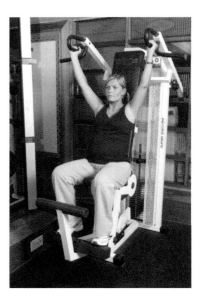

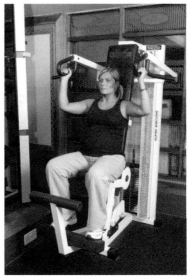

Exercises to avoid now that you are pregnant

Seated abdominal machine

While it is OK to use this machine for the first 12 weeks of your pregnancy if you used it before becoming pregnant. There are many more functional and valuable abdominal exercises you can do (see pages 31–8 in Chapter 6, which deals with core stability). Don't use this machine if you are unfamiliar with it.

Once you reach your second trimester you should stop using this machine and do some of the core stability exercises mentioned in this book instead (see pages 35–41).

Seated back extensor machine

While it is OK to use this machine for the first 12 weeks of your pregnancy if you used it before becoming pregnant. There are many more functional and valuable back exercises you can do, even when you are not pregnant (again, see pages 31–8 in Chapter 6, which deals with core stability). Don't use this machine if you are unfamiliar with it.

Once you reach your second trimester you should stop using this machine and do some of the core stability exercises mentioned in this book instead (see pages 35–41).

Seated rotation machine

While it is OK to use this machine for the first 12 weeks of your pregnancy, there are many more functional and valuable abdominal exercises you can do, even when you are not pregnant!

Once you reach your second trimester, and preferably before this point, you should stop using this machine and do some of the core stability exercises mentioned in this book instead (see pages 35–41).

Side bends

Using weights for this exercise is not ideal if you are pregnant. You can do controlled lateral flexion (side-bending movements) but should not use weights as this will stress the abdominal area, and the work on the obliques may contribute to abdominal muscle separation.

Points to remember

- If any of the exersises hurt you, feel uncomfortable or you struggle to maintain good technique, then adapt or alter the exercise.
- Remember to reduce the amount of weight used as your pregnancy progresses.
- With a low-risk pregnancy there is no reason why you can't use weights throughout your pregnancy.
- Appropriate and regular weight training will help you to maintain good tone and strength, which will help see you through the coming months and the delivery at the end of your exciting journey.
- If you are a beginner, never start weight training without expert supervision.

15. Body-conditioning and weights classes

Body-conditioning classes may be worth considering if you are keen to maintain your muscle tone during pregnancy. Not only are they a great way of keeping you well conditioned they are a brilliant way to socialise. Many people find that they are more motivated in a class situation and that they benefit from being observed and guided by the teacher. In addition, the fact that the class is at the same time and in the same place each week encourages you to keep that time-slot free and can help discipline you to attend each week.

With a low-risk pregnancy you can continue to participate in most conditioning classes if you already attended them before becoming pregnant. You will, however, have to make adaptations to the exercises involved as your pregnancy progresses (see the suggestions below).

If you are new to exercise I would suggest that you join a class that is aimed at pregnant women. If such a class is not available to you, then look for a beginners' conditioning class such as thighs, tums and bums (TTBs) or a beginners' stability ball class. I suggest, too, that you go and talk to the teachers and see if they are happy for you to attend. It is always a good idea to watch a class first before joining in.

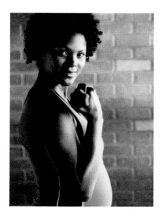

Considerations

- Make sure your teacher knows you are pregnant and feels confident enough to work with you.
- Avoid exercises that involve lying on your tummy as soon as this becomes uncomfortable.
- After 12 weeks, reduce the amount of work you do lying on your back. Omit lying on your back after 20 weeks.
- Avoid standing still for long periods.
- Avoid doing movements that involve holding your arms above your head for long periods.
- Avoid any fast, jerky movements.
- Maintain control of your movements and avoid using momentum.
- Avoid upside-down positions and positions that feel as if they crowd the uterus.
- See the guidelines on flexibility in Chapter 17.

Spotting a good teacher

- Does the teacher chat to new people and ask whether anyone is injured, pregnant, and so on?
- Is it really a beginners' class?
- Does the teacher observe class members and correct them if necessary, or do they simply shout out instructions without teaching you anything about the exercise, how to do it properly and what it is aiming to achieve?
- Does the teacher offer harder and easier options?
- Does the teacher move around the room to observe people?
- Does the teacher correct both the group as a whole and individuals?

You may find that a teacher is reluctant to take you into their class if they have never taught you before and you are pregnant. Please respect this decision as they may not feel experienced enough to deal with your specific condition.

Exercise adaptations

The following are some useful adaptations to the kinds of exercises you are likely to encounter in an average body-conditioning class. The teacher may suggest that you try these (or their own variations) but, if not, you may wish to discuss the following adaptations with them.

0–12 weeks: bench press flat on step
12–20 weeks: bench inclined, lighter weight
20–28 weeks: bench inclined, using dumbbells
28–40 weeks: bench inclined, using lighter dumbbells with somebody passing weights

0–12 weeks: sit-ups
12–20 weeks: pelvic tilts
20–28 weeks: all-fours 'Superman's
28–40 weeks: all-fours pinpoint

0–12 weeks: sit-up twist
12–20 weeks: kneeling side bends
20–28 weeks: seated side bends
28–40 weeks: all-fours hip swings

0–12 weeks: back extensions on the floor
12–28 weeks: seated hip-hinge on a stability ball
28–40 weeks: cat stretch

0–12 weeks: wide squats with bar behind neck
12–20 weeks: narrow squats with bar behind neck
20–28 weeks: narrow squats with dumbbells
28–40 weeks: dead lift with light bar

0–12 weeks: adductor lifts, leg behind body
12–28 weeks: adductor lifts with top knee on pillow
28–40 weeks: adductor squeezes with chi ball* between legs

(* A chi ball is much smaller than a stability ball. Chi balls are likely to be available for use at your gym, so ask an instructor to point one out to you.)

Studio weight-training classes

These classes (sometimes known as 'Bodypump' or 'Bodymax') are conditioning classes where weights are used. The techniques used are very different from one type of class to another. It is important you tell your instructor that you are pregnant and to ask if they are comfortable with you being in their class.

These classes are a great way to really tone and strengthen your muscles, however they are not a suitable form of exercise to start in your pregnancy. Those of you who are used to doing weight-training classes will already have worked on strengthening the bones, tendons, ligaments and muscles used in the exercises; you can continue to do these classes but will need to make adaptations as your pregnancy progresses. Towards the end of your pregnancy you may find the speed of the class too fast. If so, switch to doing the same exercises in the gym so that you can work at your own pace and speed.

Table 15.1 Weight-training class advice for each trimester

Stage of pregnancy	Weight-training class advice
1st trimester **0–12** WEEKS	• As long as you are used to these types of classes you can continue to do them as normal during your first 12 weeks of pregnancy as long as yours is a low-risk pregnancy.
1st stage of 2nd trimester **12–20** WEEKS	• From 11–20 weeks, slightly incline the step for any exercise that involves you lying flat on your back. • Avoid doing any sit-up type activities. • Avoid having a heavy barbell behind your neck after 12 weeks; reduce the amount of weight used.
2nd stage of 2nd trimester **20–28** WEEKS	• At 20–28 weeks, switch from using a barbell to dumbbells. • After 20 weeks, or sooner if necessary, avoid any exercises that involve you lying on your back. • Avoid using a barbell behind your neck after 20 weeks; switch to dumbbells. • After 20 weeks, avoid doing lunges where you step out and back; switch to split lunges where you work on the spot. • After 20 weeks, avoid exercises where the barbell or dumbbells are lifted over the head.
3rd trimester **28–40** WEEKS	• At 28–40 weeks, take extra care getting up and down from the step, and get somebody to pass you the weights.

In general...

- Avoid exercises lying on your tummy once this becomes uncomfortable.
- Reduce the number of weights you do (for *all* exercises) as your pregnancy progresses.
- When you are taking a break (or if there is no adaptation available), use the time to rest and sip water, but keep moving your feet; you could always do the foot pedals exercise described in the next chapter (page 130) or some pelvic floor work.
- Be extra vigilant with regard to your technique.
- Avoid swinging or flinging the weights, or using momentum rather than control to lift them.
- As your pregnancy progresses, gradually reduce the weight used.
- Work on an inclined bench after 12 weeks, and incline the bench further after 20 weeks.

16. Pilates

Pilates literally strengthens from the inside out, focusing on the deeper stabilising muscles. While Pilates does not have a cardiovascular training effect, it can make a marked contribution to your posture and ability to function 'normally' throughout your pregnancy. It can also help you to deal with the stresses and strains that pregnancy can place on both the body and the mind.

What is Pilates?

Pilates helps build the deep postural muscles of your trunk and spine, giving you better posture and improving core stability. It works on developing correct movement patterns in the way we walk, bend, move and sit, thus helping to prevent injury and improving your overall posture and alignment. Pilates promotes muscle balance, muscle endurance and flexibility through a series of progressive and functional exercises.

Many Pilates exercises would be considered highly controversial during pregnancy, however there are many others that are ideal for helping you develop better core stability and a stronger centre that will help support your growing baby and could help decrease the likelihood of back pain.

In a good Pilates class the pelvic floor will be addressed as will shoulder and pelvic stability, which all help to create a strong 'trunk'. If this type of exercise is followed both before and during pregnancy it can have positive effect on you in terms of reducing back pain and improving your posture and pelvic floor function.

Choosing the right Pilates class

Not all Pilates is the same. The most important thing to look for when choosing a Pilates class is an experienced teacher who is happy to work with pregnant women. Below is a list of key points to look out for when identifying a good Pilates class.

- A class should have a maximum of 12–15 participants.
- Classes should be graded: beginners, improvers, intermediate, and so on.
- Classes should be run in a course-type format. For example, a six- or ten-week course. At 'drop-in' classes, it is likely that either the experienced clients won't progress or any beginners present won't understand the concepts involved.
- You should be asked to complete a written consent form before you start your session (this is sometimes known as a 'screening form' and will ask questions relating to your health and well-being, as well as requesting details of your pregnancy).
- Look for a class that has full-length mats, pillows and blocks that can be used to help you feel comfortable and that allow exercises to be adapted to suit the individual.
- Your teacher should move around the room – and you should expect to be offered some hands-on guidance.

In general, Pilates courses are the best way to learn about this exercise method, as it is not something that you can get the hang of in just one lesson or by watching a video, say. Courses also allow the instructor to work with you on specific issues or problems you may have, and mean that you are guaranteed teacher continuity. You may find, however, that specifically pre-natal Pilates classes don't ask you to sign up for a full course as the instructor is aware that you may not always be able to make a session due to hospital appointments, and so on.

Why is Pilates good for you in pregnancy?

Pregnancy is well known as a cause of back pain, and regular and appropriate Pilates exercise may help you to reduce the risk of this. Appropriate Pilates exercise may also aid in recovery from back pain. Pilates can help to improve or maintain good posture, and help you to avoid the postural problems often associated with neck tension and headaches.

Appropriate Pilates exercise will also help to condition the deep abdominals, which will help you carry the weight of your baby. These muscles will also be used to help you in delivery and Pilates class attendance is likely to help you get your abdomen back in shape after pregnancy.

Many Pilates exercises can help increase bone density and aid the prevention of osteoporosis.

The very nature of Pilates means that you have to focus on your mind and body; this promotes relaxation and eases stress-related conditions.

As Pilates focuses on the core stabilising muscles it can also help improve the function of the pelvic floor. A beginners' course (following the guidelines above) would be an ideal form of activity for those of you who are pregnant and not already following a programme of activity. It would also be good for those of you who are already fit but want to supplement your current training programme with activity that will focus on your core stability and posture during your pregnancy. You may even find that doing Pilates later in the evening may help you to relax and sleep. Do remember, however, that not all Pilates classes are the same. Follow the guidelines above when looking for a class and ensure that you get your GP's permission if you are new to this or any other form of exercise.

Once you have found your Pilates class and are attending it regularly, you may find that it becomes more difficult after approximately 20 weeks of pregnancy, as you will no longer be able to lie on your tummy or be able to exercise for any length of time (if at all) on your back. After approximately 20 weeks you could invest in some one-to-one Pilates training or look for a teacher who is specifically qualified in pre-natal exercise as he or she will be able to make all the necessary adaptations to your Pilates programme. You may even be lucky enough to find a specific pre-natal Pilates class.

Pilates breathing

Pilates uses a method of breathing referred to as *lateral breathing* (this is where you breathe into the sides and back of the ribs – your instructor will be able to explain it to you if necessary). This is very often the principle of Pilates that people find the hardest to master and it does take time! However, as your pregnancy develops (during the latter half of the second trimester and throughout the third trimester) you may find it easier to get to grips with Pilates breathing, as you will naturally use a lateral breathing pattern. (See Chapter 3 for information about respiration and changes to the respiratory system during pregnancy).

I feel it is worth noting, however, that particularly in pregnancy it is inappropriate to get groups of people to breathe in and out at the same time. If you are 20 weeks pregnant you will breathe at a different rate to a woman who is 32 weeks pregnant. She in turn will breathe at a different rate to someone who is 40 weeks pregnant. While doing Pilates, breathe with a lateral breath but do not try to breathe at a set tempo with the rest of the group. A good Pilates teacher will set you off with an exercise then ask you to carry on at your own speed and pace, which may mean that what you are doing differs from what the person next to you is doing. This will allow you to match the pace of your exercise with the pace of your breathing. In Pilates you are encouraged to use lateral breathing in order to work the lungs effectively. It is worth mentioning, though, that Pilates is not a form of cardiovascular exercise, so it should not be necessary for you to take deep breaths throughout the class.

Because I will not be with you when you exercise, I can only encourage you to breathe normally as you do the exercises described below. Above all, avoid holding your breath. If you attend a Pilates class, however, then you can expect to be taught correct breathing technique.

Pilates programming

If you are new to Pilates you should start with a complete beginners' Pilates class with a good teacher, and possibly stay with either beginners, or improvers, Pilates throughout your pregnancy. Alternatively, look for a specific pre-natal Pilates class. For those of you who have a low-risk pregnancy and are already used to Pilates, you should be able to carry on as normal throughout the first trimester of your pregnancy. After that you will need to plan a programme of exercise that is appropriate for your needs while pregnant, and that deals with the physical limitations that pregnancy can bring.

I have listed some recommendations in Table 16.1 that may help both you and your Pilates instructor to plan appropriate exercises for you as your pregnancy progresses.

Table 16.1 Pilates class advice for each trimester

Stage of pregnancy	General pilates advice
1st trimester **0–12 WEEKS**	• Normal Pilates exercises can be continued with a low-risk pregnancy and without any increased pain. Small classes and individual observation and correction are important. If you are not already doing so, incorporate specific pelvic floor exercises into the class. Take the principles of Pilates into your everyday life. Be particularly aware of correct lifting technique and correct posture throughout your normal everyday activities. • If you are about to start a beginners' Pilates class, check to see if the teacher restricts participant numbers and works on a course basis. The teacher should ask you about your medical history, and so on, before you start the class. You must inform them that you are pregnant. If you are new to the class and the Pilates instructor does not speak to you individually then perhaps it would be best to look for a different teacher.
1st stage of 2nd trimester **12–20 WEEKS**	• Due to the fact that diastasis can occur (see pages 28–9) avoid any activity that directly works the rectus abdominis and external obliques (e.g. activities where the head and shoulders, or both knees, are lifted off the floor). • Pay specific attention to transitions when getting up from and down to the floor, and when moving from one position to another. • Gradually reduce the number of reps you do, and reduce the leverage and intensity of some of the moves as your body changes shape and your centre of gravity alters. • Avoid Pilates exercises where you have to hold one position for any length of time as this may increase your blood pressure. • Avoid direct work on the lumbar back extensors (the lower back) in the concentric phase (i.e. when the muscles are shortened as they contract); the lumbar extensors will start to shorten as your pregnancy progresses, due to postural changes. • Avoid lying on your tummy in a prone position once this becomes uncomfortable. • If you have any symptoms of supine hypotensive syndrome (see pages 165–6) then, after 12 weeks, avoid any exercises that involve lying on your back.
2nd stage of 2nd trimester **20–28 WEEKS**	• Due to supine hypotensive syndrome, the amount of time spent lying on your back should be reduced or omitted. It is important you read the section on supine hypotensive syndrome (pages 165–6) to make sure you understand the signs and symptoms. If you do have any symptoms you should not lie on your back for any length of time. • Avoid any activity that takes the legs into a wide position. • Avoid holding positions where the muscles are stretched for long periods of time. Start to work on maintaining your flexibility and avoid developmental stretches for improving flexibility. • Avoid Pilates exercises such as the full roll-down. This exercise is fine when taken to the base of the shoulder blades but may stress the lumbar spine if you bend into the lower part of the spine as your abdominals will become stretched and thus offer less support to the spine.

Stage of pregnancy	General pilates advice
1st stage of 3rd trimester **28–36** WEEKS	• By this stage it is likely that your abdominals will have started to gap, if they have not already done so. If they have, then the gap may now be getting bigger. Pilates exercises on all-fours at this stage of pregnancy are ideal, however if you are suffering from carpal tunnel syndrome you will need to make adaptations to any exercises that call for the all-fours position. • As your pregnancy progresses there is more chance of you being affected by supine hypotensive syndrome (see pages 165–6) due to the increasing size and weight of your growing baby. Omit any exercises that involve lying on your back. • Ensure that you do not stand still for any length of time. • Avoid holding positions for long periods of time. • Increase the amount of relaxation and rest between exercises and practise sustaining positions, which may be used for delivery (ask your instructor for more information about these).
2nd stage of 3rd trimester **36–40** WEEKS	• Allow plenty of time for rest and the weight literally being taken off your feet. This is an ideal time to look for a specific pre-natal class if you haven't already done so. • You can continue with Pilates at a level that feels comfortable for you even at this stage of your pregnancy. I do suggest, however, that you follow a programme that is designed specifically for pregnant women and find either a specific video or qualified pre- and post-natal Pilates teacher. • Always take particular care when getting up from and down to the floor. You should be doing some standing Pilates-based exercise to help you in your everyday life and in labour. • Reduce the length of time spent on each Pilates exercise. Continue to reduce both the number of reps and the intensity of moves, as well as the length of time for which positions are held. • Take care when moving from one position to another. • You may now find a full hour of Pilates difficult and may prefer to do shorter sessions or to exercise on alternate days. Continue, however, to do regular pelvic floor exercises. • If you find a whole class of Pilates too much then try doing shorter periods of exercise or see if your instructor will do a private 30-minute session just for you. You may, however, feel comfortable enough to continue with your specially adapted Pilates class right through to the end of your pregnancy; this will be of great benefit to you and your body now, during delivery and after the birth.

Learning good posture for later pregnancy

As your pregnancy progresses, your centre of gravity will change. This is due to the increasing size of the uterus and foetus. The curve in your lower back is likely to become more pronounced as your pelvis tilts forwards a little to accommodate your baby. However, if it is not properly managed, or if your core muscles are a little weak and underused, this curve can become excessive. Strain will be placed on your muscles in all the wrong places – in short, it will mean that you can develop a muscle imbalance in the lower body, which can contribute to back pain now and in the future.

The increased weight of your breasts may also increase the chances of your upper back becoming more rounded, increasing tightness across your pectoral (chest) muscles, and weakening your upper back.

Be aware that many standing Pilates-based exercises are very good for you in pregnancy, but you must avoid standing still for long periods of time as this can exaggerate any tendency towards poor posture. The added weight, hormonal effects and changes in the centre of gravity all mean that standing for too long can increase the strain on the lumbar spine and abdominal area; they can also cause pooling of blood in the legs, increasing the likelihood of varicose veins. At worst, the effects may even cause you to faint.

As the normal lumbar curve increases in pregnancy, optimal posture for exercising, lifting or standing should slightly lengthen the spine. This, combined with abdominal hollowing, will help you to reduce the lumbar extension and bring your spine into a more neutral 'normal' curve. These principles are of paramount importance in Pilates and that is why appropriate Pilates exercises are so useful in pregnancy.

Sample Pilates exercises suitable for use during pregnancy

The exercises on the following pages are examples of Modern Pilates that will be beneficial for you during pregnancy, even if you have not done Pilates before. They are just a selection, as there are many more than we have room for in this book.

Shoulder shrugs

Purpose

- To relax the muscles between the shoulders and the back of the neck (upper trapezius)
- To exercise the muscles that help to stabilise the shoulder blades (lower trapezius and serratus anterior)
- To allow you to find your correct shoulder position

Start position

- You can do this exercise seated or standing
- Keep your feet hip with apart (sit on your 'sitting bones' if seated), hands down in line with your hips, pelvis and spine in neutral, knees relaxed

Action

- Engage your abdominals by pulling your tummy in towards your spine slightly
- Shrug your shoulders up by your ears for a count of two
- Slowly lower your shoulders and continue to draw your shoulder blades down your back for a count of four.

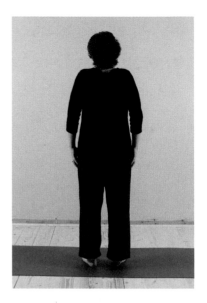

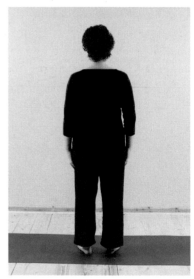

Arm floats

Purpose

- To improve your shoulder and trunk stability

Start position

- You can do this exercise seated or standing
- Keep your feet hip width apart (sit on your 'sitting bones' if seated), hands down in line with your hips, pelvis and spine in neutral, knees relaxed

Action

- Engage your abdominals by pulling your tummy towards your spine slightly
- Draw your shoulder blades down the spine (do not squeeze them together – draw them down)
- Allow your shoulder blades to stay drawn down and flat to your rib cage as you 'float' your arms forwards up to shoulder height
- Maintain the space between your shoulders and ears – don't lift your shoulders as you lift your arms
- The arms should feel light, elbows soft – as if holding a big balloon
- Ensure that, as your arms lift, there is no movement in the lower back, and avoid leaning backwards
- Lower the arms and repeat

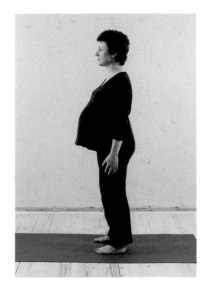

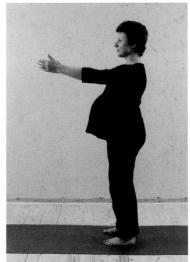

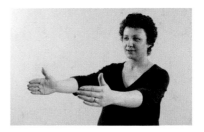

Foot pedals

Avoid this exercise if it increases or causes any pain in the front or back of the pelvis.

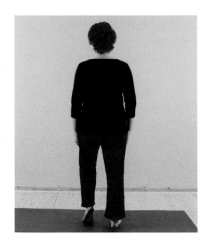

Purpose

- To improve the stability of your pelvis, as well as your core stability, general circulation, balance and coordination.
- To improve ankle mobility

Start position

- Keep your feet and knees hip distance apart, keep the knees relaxed (but not bent), shoulders down away from your ears
- Point your fingers down your sides as if in line with the side seam of a pair of trousers
- Keep the back of your neck long, with the crown of your head towards the ceiling
- The base of your spine (sacrum) should be lengthened towards the floor

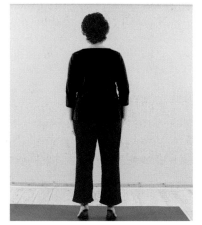

Action

- Engage your abdominals by pulling your tummy towards your spine slightly
- Peel one heel up off the floor, taking the weight into the ball of the foot
- Return the foot down to the floor and repeat on the opposite foot
- Make sure your pelvis does not rock from side to side
- Once you have got used to this, then start to 'pedal' your feet – as one heel is coming down the other heel is lifting up, switching from foot to foot; the knee is allowed to bend while the top of the pelvis should stay level and still
- Repeat several times

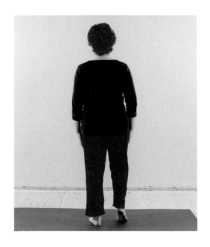

Tip

As your pregnancy reaches full term you will need to ensure that your pelvis is able to stay still and, if necessary, hold on to something just lightly to help you balance. Make sure you use something that does not make you lean forwards, though.

Dumb waiter

Purpose

- To open up the muscles across the front of your chest and the front of your shoulders, while strengthening your shoulder retractors (which are in between your shoulder blades)

Start position

- As for foot pedals, above; you can also do this exercise seated

Action

- Engage your abdominals by pulling your tummy towards your spine
- Ensure the lumbar spine stays in its neutral position and that your chin stays softly nodded down towards your chest, ears in line with your shoulders, back of your neck lengthened
- The movement should come from the upper back, not the mid- or lower back
- Palms facing up to the ceiling, elbows bent, staying close to the lower ribs
- Take your forearms out to the side and backwards, leading the movement with the thumbs as if you are forming a crease between your shoulder blades
- Abdominals stay hollowed, the shoulders stay drawn down the back and the elbows stay tucked into the body
- Release back to the start position

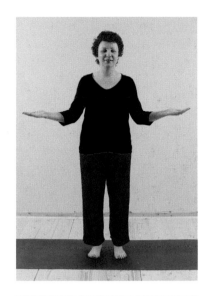

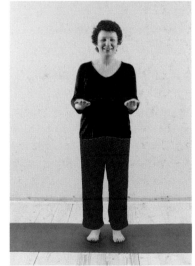

Level 2: pinpoint position

- Start position as for all-fours abdominal hollowing, above
- Draw the shoulders away from your ears; think of bringing your elbows in towards your ribs, head in line and spine in neutral
- Ensure that your spine stays in neutral and your abdominals hollowed (drawing your hip bones closer together)
- Lengthen your right arm out in front of your body at shoulder height, touching your fingers on the floor
- Your shoulders should stay level – avoid reaching forwards
- Take your left leg out behind your body, touching the floor with your toes
- Your hips should stay level
- Keep your body in line and hold for a few seconds, breathing normally
- Bring your hand and leg back in line and repeat on the opposite side
- Your abdominals should stay hollowed throughout; also, keep your shoulders stabilised and drawn down
- Sit back and rest your wrists if you need to
- Repeat three to four times on each side

Level 3: 'Superman'

- Keeping your head in line with your spine, hollow your abdominals keeping your spine in neutral
- As above, opposite arm and leg 'pinpointed' on the floor
- Lift your left hand up in line with your shoulder, leading with the thumb
- Hold for a few seconds and return to the pinpoint position
- Lift your leg off the floor, maintaining your pelvis in a flat position, leg straight
- Hold for a few seconds and then return to the start position
- Repeat on the opposite side
- Do two to four reps on each side

Side leg series

Purpose

- To strengthen the deep muscles around the abdomen and back; this exercise focuses on pelvic stability and will tone the muscles in the outside of the hip and thigh

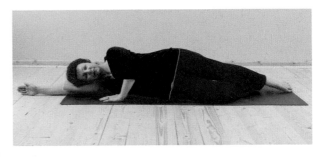

Start position

- Lay on one side, supporting your head on your arm (use a block under your head if necessary, and keep your arm out in front of your body if you have a shoulder injury); line your body up: hips and shoulders stacked, weight on your supporting hand in front of you, balanced on the block if used, toes slightly in front of your shoulders

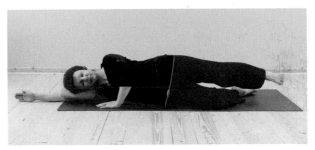

Action

- Draw your baby towards your spine – feel as if you are lifting your bottom rib 1 mm off the floor
- Lift your top leg so that it is in line with the top of your hip
- Maintain the space between your hip and rib; your pelvis should stay still as you lift your leg
- Flex your foot, bringing your toes towards your shin, and then lower your leg, continuing to lengthen your leg as you lower it
- Repeat 6–12 times on each leg

17. Flexibility and yoga during pregnancy

Some of you may be familiar with flexibility work, and already incorporate in into your everyday fitness programme. Sometimes you may feel so tired (especially in the early and late stages of your pregnancy) that a bit of gentle stretching is all you feel up to. Stretching is a great way to get rid of aches and pains and lift your spirits, but it is often the part of any fitness programme that gets neglected. However, it is a fantastic complement to any cardiovascular and conditioning exercises you do.

We have already looked at the importance of keeping your muscles toned and strong to help you maintain good posture during pregnancy. Stretching can prevent your muscles from becoming tight and can also help relieve tension and pain. However, you must be aware of your own limitations when stretching in pregnancy. I have already mentioned the effects of relaxin (see page 9), a hormone that relaxes your ligaments and tendons during pregnancy, making your joints unstable. While this is essential for birth, it means that you have to be extra careful when stretching. In pregnancy there is the risk of overstretching, as you will be able to get into positions that you weren't able to previously. Maybe you couldn't do the

---

Stretching essentials

The following guidelines should help you to stretch safely.

- Whenever you stretch ensure that you feel balanced and supported
- Avoid lying on your back to stretch after 20 weeks
- Stretch so you can feel a lengthening in the muscle but avoid stretching to your maximum
- Never bounce when you stretch
- Breathe normally as you stretch; avoid holding your breath
- Avoid holding stretches for long periods of time
- Avoid stretches where the muscle is stretched, then contracted then stretched further (these are known as PNF stretches – ask your gym instructor for more information about these if necessary)
- You should feel tension as you stretch, never pain

splits before you were pregnant but feel you may be able to now – *don't*! If you overstretch your ligaments they may stay that way and, long after your baby is born, you may suffer from unstable joints and, eventually, injury. The main thing to remember is to stretch *slowly* and *gently*.

When to stretch

As a teacher trainer for the YMCA I used to recommend that stretches were included in the warm-up for most activities. However, recent research has placed a question mark over the effectiveness of stretching during warm-up. I agree that in many activities where the muscles are not excessively stressed or taken beyond a normal range of movement stretching is not always necessary. When we exercise in pregnancy, and specifically after the first trimester, we want to exercise in a non-maximal way, and we do not want to use excessive ranges of motion, as our joints and the like are unstable. I do not feel, however, that doing short static stretches (between 8 and 10 seconds) will do you any harm as long as they are specifically designed for your stage of pregnancy. Although, if you don't stretch at the start of your warm-up, don't worry, you won't be arrested by the 'do it right' police!

So, to conclude, I don't give specific warm-up stretches in this book, for the reasons outlined above. However if you do go into an exercise session and feel that your muscles are tight or you have a lot of tension, then go ahead: warm up your muscles first and then do any stretches you feel are necessary, using this chapter for reference.

Stretches at the end of your workout

In most types of workout you would benefit from some sort of a stretch at the end of your session. Stretching will help your body to return to its pre-exercise state (only more refreshed, relaxed and fitter). Some schools of thought say that stretching at the end of a workout session may help offset muscle soreness (unless you have overdone things, then you will have muscle soreness whether you stretch or not). Stretching will also prevent your muscles from becoming short and tight, promoting instead length and flexibility. Stretching at the end of your session can help facilitate muscle repair, aid prevention of injury and ease tension.

You can stretch every day for a few minutes if you follow the guidelines above and in Table 17.1.

Stretches to avoid in pregnancy

- Splits
- Hurdle stretch
- Crab stretch
- Down dog (unless experienced)
- Up dog
- Abdominal stretches
- The plough
- Touching the toes standing
- Touching the toes seated
- Flinging arms back
- Flinging body side to side

Table 17.1 Stretching advice for each trimester

Stage of pregnancy	Stretching advice
1st trimester **0–12** WEEKS	You can stretch as normal (unless you have hyper-flexible joints) during your first trimester.
1st stage of 2nd trimester **12–20** WEEKS	You can stretch as normal, but avoid the stretches mentioned in the box above. Start to reduce what are known as the 'developmental stretches' (those where you hold the stretch before taking it further, gradually increasing the intensity).
2nd stage of 2nd trimester **20–28** WEEKS	Avoid stretches lying on your back. Avoid developmental stretches (as mentioned above) and avoid holding stretches for more than 30 seconds. Adjust the stretches so that you feel balanced and your pelvis feels supported.
3rd trimester **28–40** WEEKS	See above. Avoid wide-leg stretches if you have any pain down the front or back of your pelvis. Pay specific attention to stretching your hip flexors (the muscles that connect the thigh to the pelvis), chest muscles and hamstrings as these tend to get tight towards the end of pregnancy.

Calf stretch

This is a good stretch to do if you get cramp in the lower leg.

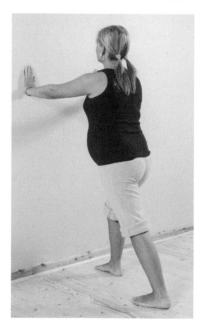

- Stand facing a wall, with the palms of your hands against it. Take your right leg forwards and your left leg back. Make sure both feet are pointing forwards. Keep your spine in alignment as you lean forwards and draw the baby towards your spine.
- Bend your front leg until you feel a stretch in the calf of your back leg.
- Breathe normally throughout the stretch and hold for 8–12 seconds on each leg.

Hamstring stretch

- Sit on a chair or, even better, a stability ball.
- Feet and knees hip distance apart, maintain good spine alignment and draw the baby close to your spine. Straighten your right leg out in front of you with the foot down. Tilt your pelvis behind you, lengthening your spine as you keep your hands on your left knee and lean forwards until you feel a stretch in the hamstring at the back of your leg.
- Breathe normally throughout the stretch and hold for 8–12 seconds on each leg.

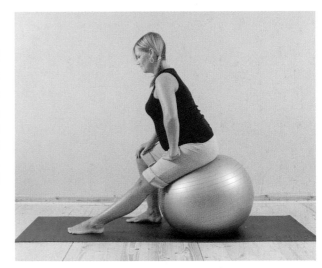

Quadriceps (quad) stretch

This stretch aims to lengthen the quadriceps muscle at the front of the thigh.

- Lie down on your right-hand side with your head supported on your arm. Bend your knees in front of you. Bring your left foot behind you towards your buttocks, keeping the knee in line with the hip, and grab hold of your foot with your left hand.
- As you pull your foot in towards your left buttock cheek (being careful to leave a small gap), gently press your left hip forwards, simultaneously drawing the baby towards your spine.
- Avoid lifting your knee up, bringing your leg behind you too far or arching your lower back. If you struggle to reach your foot, try putting a tie or shoelace round your ankle and holding this. Breathe normally throughout the stretch and hold for 8–12 seconds on each leg.

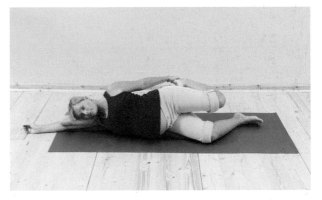

Adductor stretch

This stretch aims to lengthen the muscles on the inside of the thigh and the lower back. Do not do it if you have symphysis pubis dysfunction or feel any strain on the front of the pelvis.

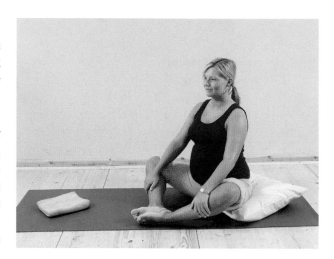

- Sit on the floor in an upright position. Bend your knees bringing the soles of your feet together, keeping the feet away from your body. Hold on to your calves. Press gently into your knees as you draw the abdominals in and round your spine forwards.
- If you find your abdominals push out then do the exercise with a straight spine.
- Breathe normally throughout the stretch and hold for 5–10 seconds.

Abductor stretch

Many of the normal abductor stretches will become difficult in the third trimester due to the size of your tummy. This exercise aims to stretch the muscles in the outside of the thigh (abductors) and the muscle deep under the buttocks (the piriformis). Do not do it if you do not have good balance. Holding on to the side of a steady armchair will help you keep your balance.

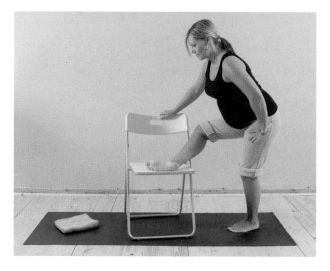

- Hold on to the chair and place the outside of your right leg on the arm of the chair. Keep your abdominals contracted as you bend your supporting leg and lean towards your right leg. Move into the stretch until you can feel mild tension.
- Breathe normally throughout the stretch and hold for eight seconds on each leg.

Hip flexor stretch

This exercise aims to stretch the muscle that attaches the thigh to the pelvis (the hip flexor). You can do this exercise kneeling or standing.

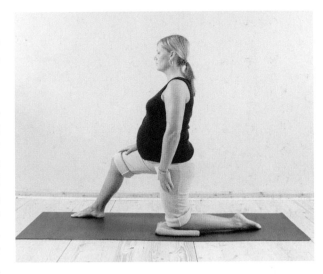

- Kneel on your left knee, place a folded towel under the knee to protect it (do the standing exercise if you have knee pain or difficulty maintaining balance and good alignment). Take your right leg out in front of you, toes pointed forwards. Ensure that you have space at the back of your right knee. Place your right hand on your right knee or on a support to the side of you. Lengthen the spine and tuck your pelvis under you, drawing the abdominals towards your spine, then move your whole body forwards slightly.
- Ensure that you do not bend forwards or arch backwards. This exercise is about trying to lengthen the hip flexor rather than move forwards.
- You may find that the standing stretch is easier to do in the third trimester.

Cat stretch

This is excellent for stretching the spine and back muscles, releasing tension and maintaining mobility in the spine (as the lower back tends to overarch during pregnancy). It will also work the abdominals in a safe, non-weight-bearing, manner.

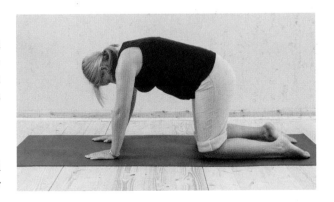

- Start in the all-fours position.
- Check that your knees are under your hips and the hands are at a slight angle in front of your shoulders.
- Keep your spine in neutral alignment (see Chapter 16, page 127) and your abdominals pulled in.
- Breathe in to the back and sides of the ribs and, as you breathe out, continue to contract your

abdominals and tuck your tailbone under you as much as you can. Lift your lower back up towards the ceiling and drop your head as if looking towards your baby.

● Hold for a few seconds as you breathe normally. As you release the spine try to use what is called segmental control (do it bit by bit) – feel as if you are lengthening the spine rather than arching upwards. Release your head and shoulders first, then your mid-spine, eventually taking the pelvis back into neutral position.

● Take the weight off your hands.

● Repeat three to five times.

This exercise can also be performed with your elbows supported on blocks or a low chair if you suffer from carpal tunnel syndrome.

Chest stretch

You need a partner to help you do this exercise. They should apply gentle pressure only, not force. It is a great way to stretch the pectoral minor (the chest muscle that does not attach directly to the humerus). After the 12th week of pregnancy prop yourself up on pillows so that your head and shoulders are lifted slightly. Avoid this stretch completely if you get any symptoms of supine hypotensive syndrome (see page 165–6).

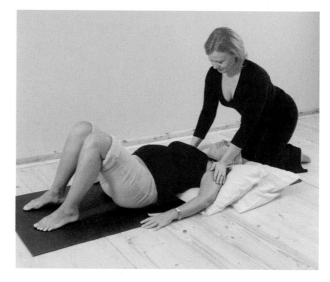

● Lie on your back with your knees bent, feet hip width apart and your arms down by the side of your body – your head should be in line with your spine (use a small pillow if necessary).

● Get your partner to kneel behind you and apply a little pressure to your shoulders (avoid letting your rib cage lift).

● Hold for eight seconds, relax, then repeat.

Triceps stretch

Again, seated is a good position for this stretch, which will help maintain flexibility in the back of the arms.

- Sit upright on the edge of a bench or on a stability ball and maintain a slight abdominal contraction throughout the exercise.
- Take one hand behind your head, elbow close to your ear, as if you are reaching for your bra strap. Place the opposite hand on the back of the arm and apply pressure until you feel a stretch in the back of the arm.
- Breathe normally throughout the exercise and hold for eight seconds.
- Repeat on the other side.

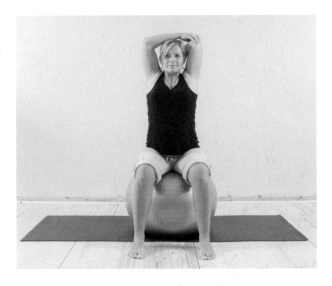

Side stretch 1

This is a good stretch for the waist and spinal muscles. It also helps maintain mobility in the spine. Aim for a slight stretch rather than rotating as far as you can.

- Sit on the edge of a bench or on a stability ball. Maintain your spine in an upright position and draw the baby towards your back. Feel as if you are lengthening the crown of your head towards the ceiling.
- Place your right hand on your left knee and your left hand slightly behind your body. Pull on your left knee so that you twist your body to your left, lengthening your spine as you do so.
- Breathe throughout the exercise and hold for a few seconds. Do it twice on each side.

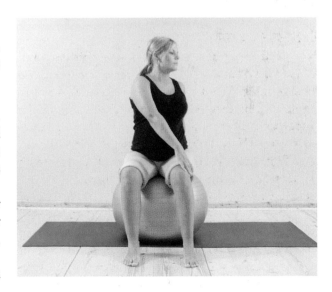

Side stretch 2

The second side stretch is great for stretching the muscles at the sides of the body but is also useful if baby's bottom (or head) is digging in to your ribs. It may also help you to breathe a little easier.

- Use a seated or standing position.
- Draw the baby towards your spine a little and lift your right arm upwards towards the ceiling. Support your body with the opposite hand either on your hip or the floor. Lift your right arm a little higher if you can, stretching to the fingertips, and lean slightly to the left.
- As you hold the position ensure that you do not arch your lower back. This sounds difficult, but try breathing into the right lung as you hold the stretch.
- Hold the stretch as you breathe in and out twice. Maintain the feeling of lengthening upwards rather than over, backwards or forwards. Hold for eight seconds then repeat on the other side. Do it twice on each side.

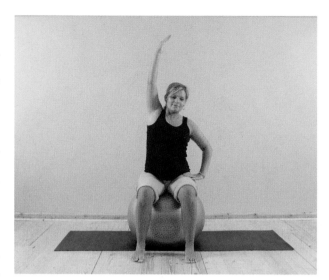

Neck stretch

This stretch aims to lengthen the muscles at the sides and back of the neck. It is a great stretch to do at your desk.

- Sit on a bench or chair, maintain an upright position and a slight abdominal contraction. Let your arms relax by your sides. Imagine you are taking your right ear up to the ceiling as you press the right shoulder down – make sure both shoulders stay level though.
- Breathe throughout the exercise and hold for eight seconds. Repeat on the opposite side.

Yoga during pregnancy

I have included yoga in this chapter on flexibility as one of the main thrusts of yoga is that it focuses on positions and movements that can improve your flexibility, so all the rules discussed above still apply.

There are many different types of yoga and many of these have become particularly popular in the past few years. Dynamic yoga is not appropriate in pregnancy unless you are very experienced in this method. Even then you will need to get specific advice from a yoga professional who is qualified in pregnancy, as you will need to adapt many moves. One of the types of yoga to become popular more recently is Bikram yoga, where you perform the positions in very hot conditions. *Do not do this type of yoga if you are pregnant or planning to get pregnant.*

You will gain much more than flexibility from yoga: it will aid balance, stability, relaxation, meditation and self-awareness. If you are used to yoga then you must tell your teacher you are pregnant and ensure that they feel knowledgeable enough to have you in their class. If they have no experience in this field it is not enough for them to say 'Take it easy' or 'Listen to your body'. You may need to look for a different or specialist teacher and your current instructor, as a professional, will probably suggest this or, at the very least, understand and respect your decision.

If you are new to yoga and pregnant, then look for a complete beginners' class with a teacher who feels comfortable working with you, or seek out a pregnancy yoga class. Yoga can be very good for you if it is specifically designed for pregnancy. Many people see yoga as a good form of exercise during pregnancy, however due to your lack of stability and lax ligaments at this time it is not ideal for you to join a mainstream yoga class if you have not been doing yoga prior to becoming pregnant.

I know many women who have done yoga throughout their pregnancies, many of them with a specifically qualified teacher, and they have found it of great benefit in helping them relax. They have even been able to use some of the breathing, meditation and relaxation techniques in labour.

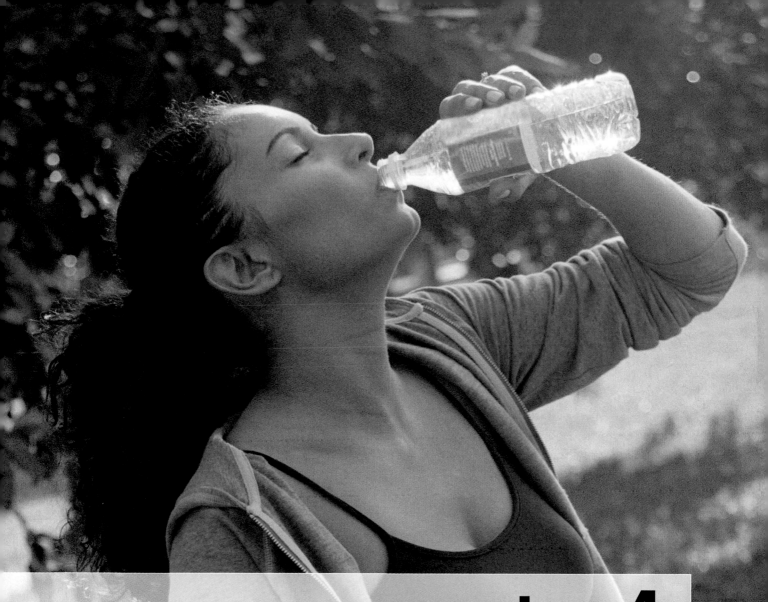

part 4

Healthy eating during pregnancy

18. The importance of eating the right foods

Taking in the right nutrients is important at any time, but never more so than when you are doing such an important job as growing another human being. Good nutrition in pregnancy can affect not only you and your health during your pregnancy, but also in the years to come. Poor nutrition in pregnancy can rob your body of essential nutrients such as calcium, making you prone to bone loss (osteoporosis) and problems with your teeth and gums. Poor nutrition while pregnant can affect your baby into its childhood; he or she may have more allergies, or be more prone to general sickness, and so on.

What you eat directly affects your growing baby. The foetus receives nutrients and oxygen direct from your bloodstream via the placenta and through the umbilical cord. Waste materials from the foetus are returned into the mother's bloodstream and will be excreted with the mother's own waste products.

A healthy, well-functioning placenta in pregnancy is therefore essential. Some mums-to-be will have problems with the placenta and may find that this affects their baby's development; while this is rare, it often has absolutely nothing to do with what they have or have not done. However, in early pregnancy, placental development is at its most critical stage and can be affected by poor nutrition, drugs or alcohol. If you have any kind of eating disorder you should seek medical advice and try to improve your nutrition, physical and mental health before you get pregnant. Being very underweight may compromise your fertility and you may find it harder to get pregnant. Being very underweight and having poor nutrition will not only affect you, it can have detrimental effects on your baby's nutrition both in the womb and in childhood. Babies born to mums who have had poor nutrition (for whatever reason) can have reduced height, dental problems, smaller brain cells and learning difficulties.

I understand that in early and late pregnancy you may feel that you spend more time in the loo than anywhere else. I also understand (and remember) how frustrating, time-consuming and inconvenient this is. Despite this, you still need to drink, otherwise you may find that not only do you get dehydrated, but your skin will suffer and you may become constipated. You may even get a urine infection, which is not good at the best of times but may be harder than usual to get rid of when you are pregnant as you can't take over-the-counter medicines. When you pee your urine should be pale. Keep an eye on this – if it isn't pale then you are not drinking enough.

19. Vitamins and minerals

With the increased demands placed on you by a growing baby, ensuring you are getting enough vitamins may not always be an easy task, but it is an important one. It is better to strive towards getting all the vitamins and minerals you need from your diet rather than from supplements. However, this may not always be possible and it is much better to take supplements than do nothing at all. However, you should only take supplements that are specifically designed for use in pregnancy and that are recommended by your GP or healthcare provider.

Vitamins

Vitamin A

Vitamin A is essential for bone and cell growth, and the development of healthy hair and nails. High levels in the body can be toxic, so avoid taking supplements containing vitamin A or ensure that you don't exceed the recommended daily amount.

Vitamin A can be found in cooked spinach, broccoli, milk, yoghurt, liver, fatty fish and brightly coloured vegetables.

Vitamins B1 and B6

Vitamin B is a water-soluble vitamin. The B vitamins are important in pregnancy as they help release energy during metabolism. They also help in maintaining healthy tissues in the body and promoting cell growth. Vitamin B1, however, can be stored in the body, so while you need to take care not to take too much of this vitamin it is important in the first and second trimesters as the foetus uses carbohydrates for development. Vitamin B1 helps metabolise carbohydrates in the body; it also helps maintain the health of your muscles, heat and nerves.

Vitamin B6 can be found in meat, chicken, fish, bananas, soya beans, green-leaf vegetables and potatoes.

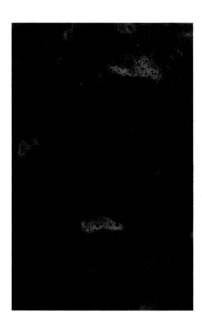

Vitamin C

Vitamin C is important in helping to maintain healthy muscles, connective tissue and bones. It is essential in forming iron from haemoglobin and red blood cells, and therefore vital in maintaining a healthy pregnancy.

Vitamin C can be found in broccoli, oranges, peppers, tomatoes and kiwi fruit.

Vitamin D

Vitamin D is essential in pregnancy for the formation and maintenance of bones, which is obviously important for baby but also matters for you too. As well as coming from your diet, vitamin D is also produced in the body as a result of exposure to the sun (although don't forget that overexposure to the sun's rays is not good for you at any time).

Vitamin D can be found in fish-liver oil, tuna, egg yolk and salmon. Exposure to sunlight can also help your body's natural production of vitamin D.

Vitamins E and K

Vitamins E and K are also important during pregnancy, but deficiencies in those eating a normal diet are rare.

Vitamin E can be found in soya beans, asparagus, nuts, fish and eggs. Vitamin K can be found in pork, dark-green leafy vegetables and oats.

Minerals

Zinc

Zinc is a mineral that maintains tissues and helps to regulate insulin activity. It is specifically important in the third trimester as it protects the immune system and promotes growth.

Zinc can be found in oysters (although it is not advisable to eat these when you are pregnant), meat, yoghurt and fortified cereals.

Calcium

Calcium is important in pregnancy as it works with vitamin D to reduce the perception of pain. It will help your baby to develop strong bones. It will also help maintain your own bone density and protect against osteoporosis (as will regular weight-bearing activity, as we have seen in this book). Calcium is also important in maintaining the health and function of the nervous system, heart and muscles. Exercise helps the body to retain calcium as well as maintain or improve bone density.

Calcium can be found in cheese, milk, yoghurt, dark-green leafy vegetables and tinned salmon (if you eat the bones).

Folic acid

Folic acid is important because it helps create the essential building blocks for your baby. It is vital to ensure that you are getting enough folic acid before you become pregnant because it is believed that taking it may prevent your baby from developing birth defects.

Folic acid can be found in broccoli, green-leaf vegetables, avocados, oranges and legumes.

Iron

Iron is important because it helps to protect against anaemia, and it helps the body to manufacture all the extra blood that you will need during pregnancy. (There is more about iron supplements on page 149 of Chapter 20, under the subheading 'Vegetarianism'.)

Iron can be found in dark-leaf vegetables, red meat, beans, lentils, eggs, bran and oatmeal.

Lack of zinc, iron and folic acid can cause anaemia: this and extreme dehydration can cause premature labour. If you are anaemic you may be prescribed iron tablets. These can cause constipation. Ensure that you drink sufficient water, and drink orange juice, too, as this contains vitamin c, which will aid in the absorption of iron. Prunes can also help. Try to ensure that you eat sufficient iron in your diet and enough vitamin C to absorb it! It is far better to increase iron in your diet than wait to be prescribed iron tablets.

If you have an iron deficiency, Mother Nature takes over and ensures that the developing baby takes priority over you for iron in the blood-stream. It is unlikely, except in extreme cases, that your baby will suffer from iron deficiency.

The symptoms of iron deficiency are outlined in the accompanying box.

My good friend Helena is an exercise teacher and is studying for her Master's in nutrition, so I accept that she is probably more in tune with her health and nutrition than most of us.

She and I were talking about nutrition in pregnancy as I was writing

Are you iron-deficient?

If you have any of the following symptoms, this may indicate that you are iron-deficient. If you are concerned about this then speak to your GP.

- Feeling exhausted
- Feeling lethargic
- Feeling breathless
- Having a pale pallor
- General weakness
- Experiencing palpitations

this book. She said that she is not a big red meat eater under normal circumstances. Yet when pregnant with her last baby (and what a real cutie she is) she ate more red meat than usual and drank glasses of fresh orange juice. Helena said that it was not a conscious thing but more of a response to how her body felt and what she felt it was asking for.

It is no surprise that as there is more blood volume in pregnancy you will need more red blood cells to maintain your haemoglobin levels. These need sufficient iron for their production. Tea and coffee can actually hinder the absorption of vitamin C; this in turn may mean that we do not absorb iron from our food. It is also worth mentioning that it can take up to six weeks to rebuild your haemoglobin levels, so don't give up on the iron in your diet, or your tablets if you feel they are not working straight away.

There is much more I could write about vitamins and minerals. I have only touched on many of the important vitamins and minerals available – there are many more that could be mentioned here. There are other books (see the Bibliography at the end of this book) that can give you more in-depth advice and guidance. Remember, however, that a good, well-balanced diet and hydration go a long way to ensuring that you have sufficient vitamins and minerals, and the odd bit of chocolate won't do you or your baby any harm!

20. Food groups

Protein

Protein is essential during pregnancy. It is important for cell growth. Need I say more?

There are 22 essential amino acids that provide us with the protein necessary for cell growth. Protein is also important for foetal brain growth in later pregnancy.

Good sources of protein are lean meat, skinless poultry, fish, eggs, nuts, beans and lentils.

Carbohydrates in pregnancy

Carbohydrates are essential energy-givers, both for you and your baby. Refined sugars and carbohydrates can give you an instant boost but this is usually followed fairly quickly by a 'crash', when your blood sugar levels drop again. Unrefined or complex carbohydrates will give you more sustained energy as they are released into your system more slowly than refined carbohydrates. Unrefined carbohydrates are foods such as whole grains, legumes, and some fruits and vegetables. Porridge is a particularly good example of slow-release, complex carbohydrate. These foods also contain more fibre than refined carbohydrates.

In the first trimester your body utilises more carbohydrate for dealing with the pregnancy. This can mean that you feel less energetic and get tired more easily. When your pregnancy reaches the second and third trimester you may feel your energy return. In the third trimester your baby uses more protein to sustain its growth and the development of its brain. It uses fewer carbohydrates, though, so there are more of these for you, which can mean more energy.

Good sources of carbohydrate are wholegrain foods, brown rice, wholemeal bread, beans, fruit and vegetables, bulgar wheat, rice and rice cakes.

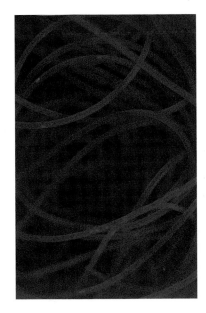

Fat

In the previous chapter, I touched on the problems of too much fat in the diet. However, some fat is 'good fat', and this sort of fat is necessary in pregnancy and everyday life. We need fat for fuel and we need to store fat for emergency use. We need fat for warmth and hormone production. We also need fat to protect our internal organs.

You may find that you deposit fat cells in your body more and in different places than you did before you were pregnant. A good diet can help you avoid laying down too much fat, although it is necessary to have some, so that your baby has sufficient fatty acids. If you eat a varied and healthy diet you can't fail to get enough fat – you may have to make an effort to eat sufficient protein or change the types of carbohydrate you eat, but you should not have any trouble ensuring you get sufficient fat. The best sources of 'good fat' are foods such as meat, eggs, fish, olives and avocados; try to avoid excessive intake of chocolate, butter, cream and cheese, although as long as you are eating a healthy, balanced diet it is OK to have these occasionally and *in moderation*.

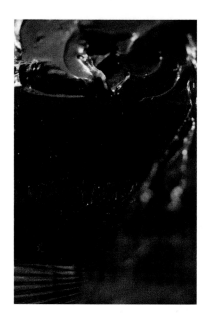

Vegetarianism

If you are a vegetarian you may find it difficult to get enough iron in your diet, particularly when you are pregnant. This is something that you will need to discuss with your GP or healthcare team, and they may recommend that you take iron supplements (see page 140 of the previous chapter, under the subheading 'Iron'). It is better to take these on a relatively empty stomach, but make sure your body is well hydrated and that you either drink some fresh orange juice at the same time or, if you can't stomach that, then take a vitamin C supplement (this is necessary because vitamin C plays an important role in iron absorption and taking the two at the same time will help you to get maximum benefit from your iron tablets). Don't take your tablets with a cup of tea or coffee, or any other drink that contains caffeine, as this will affect the vitamin C absorption. Avoid taking your tablet with milk and don't take any other vitamin supplement at the same time as your iron and vitamin C. Ensure you have your GP's approval before taking any supplements.

If you find that taking iron tablets makes you constipated, ensure that you drink plenty of water, and eat small and regular meals. Drink plenty of orange juice. Prunes can help too, as can regular exercise such as walking or swimming. If your tablets make you feel nauseous then you may have to take them with your meals. This may mean that they are not absorbed as well, but it's better than throwing them up!

Cravings

During my pregnancies I had a craving for Peking duck, but to be honest I always do! I also had a huge obsession with bleach – I could sniff it all day and have never had such a clean house. Some of you will have strange cravings during your pregnancy, but what's that got to do with exercise? To exercise – particularly when you are pregnant – you should be well hydrated and well nourished. At times, cravings are our bodies' way of telling us that we need something that is lacking in our diet, so it is always worth mentioning excessive cravings to your medical care team.

Drinks

Generally, herbal and fruit teas are known to be good for you. However, avoid drinking some of the more obscure herbal teas as some, such as devil's claw root, have been shown to cause complications in pregnancy. Drinking any herbal tea in large amounts is not recommended – try to vary the type you drink. In general, fruit teas are better than herbal teas in pregnancy, but if you have a passion for drinking anything in large amounts do check this out with your doctor.

Daily serving recommendations

- 2–3 servings of dairy products, such as milk, yoghurt or cheese; these can be from soya-based products if you wish
- 3–5 servings of mixed, coloured vegetables
- 2–4 servings of mixed, coloured fruit
- 5–7 servings of rice, pasta, cereals or bread
- 3–5 servings of protein, meat, fish, poultry, beans, nuts or eggs

Making the best choice for you and your baby
- Grain pulses (carbohydrates): choose wholegrain and enriched products wherever possible.
- Vegetables and fruit: choose dark-green and orange vegetables, and orange fruit wherever possible.
- Milk products: choose lower-fat milk products wherever possible.

Foods to avoid

- During pregnancy (and at any other time, come to think of it) avoid high intakes of high-cholesterol and high-fat foods
- You should also avoid caffeine and alcohol, and don't smoke!
- Avoid non-prescription drugs and, when being prescribed medication, don't forget to ask your GP if it's OK for you to take during pregnancy
- Avoid vitamin A supplements
- Avoid raw eggs
- Avoid raw and smoked animal foods
- Avoid oysters, raw fish and sushi
- Avoid rare-cooked meat
- Avoid paté

● Meat and alternatives (protein): choose leaner meats, poultry and fish, as well as dried peas, beans and lentils wherever possible.

What's in a serving?

Obsession with any one thing is never a good idea – and that applies to food intake too! Constantly counting calories and measuring amounts can be a bit obsessive; it is also boring and time-consuming. I am sure that every one of you reading this book has better things to do with your time. For this reason, and because I believe in making life easier wherever possible, I have tried to give you a quick and easy guide to how much is in a serving (see below). Note, however, that these guidelines are approximate.

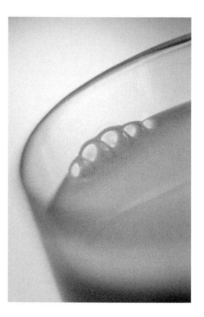

One serving of protein =
● 3.5 oz chicken, meat, fish (generally the size of your palm)
● 2 slices of cheese
● 2 eggs, 1 cup of beans, handful of nuts, 3 cups of soya milk, 1 whole-milk yoghurt, 2 tablespoons of peanut butter

One serving of dairy =
● 1 average yoghurt (175 gm)
● 1 cup milk

One serving of vegetables and fruit =
● 1 medium-sized piece of fruit or vegetable
● half a cup of frozen or canned fruit or vegetables
● half a cup of fresh fruit or vegetable juice
● 1 cup of mixed salad

One serving of carbohydrates =
● 1 slice of wholemeal bread
● 1 cup of cereal
● 1 bagel
● 1 pitta bread
● 1 cup of pasta or rice

For good health in your pregnancy...

Maintain a varied diet, using the guidelines in this book to ensure that you are taking in sufficient nutrients and calories. Avoid caffeine.

Reduce fats and simple sugars during pregnancy. Depending on your normal daily food intake, you may need to increase the amount of protein, complex carbohydrates and fibre you take in. Eat foods that are rich in vitamins and minerals, and don't forget to stay well hydrated (water is always the best bet for this).

The end result

While this book includes lots of information about exercise and diet in pregnancy in particular, you should also carry the practices described through to your everyday, non-pregnant life too. Think about how you get in and out of a chair and how you get in and out of the car or the bath. Take your time when getting up and down or moving from one position to another. When you lift or carry anything, use the techniques described in this book (see, for instance, the monkey squat on page 132).

   Remember: never be afraid or too proud to ask for help. You will be amazed at how hard normally simple everyday tasks can get – even putting your knickers on eventually becomes a feat akin to climbing Mount Everest!

   I hope this book will be of use to you. Many of you will have followed a sensible well-balanced diet, and exercised regularly and often at an appropriate level throughout your pregnancy. Some of you will have a neat little bump and will only put on weight in the right places; others of you – like me and many others – may be considerably bigger. It is not the aim of this book to keep us all looking like supermodels: you're pregnant and should look like you are! Some of you may have bottoms of steel, while others, despite some effort, may feel like your bottom is far from the same one you had nine months ago. Well it's your bottom, it's a pregnant bottom and it's a beautiful bottom, and what you will have if you follow the advice in this book is great circulation, core muscles to be proud of, posture to write home about and a pelvic floor that is the envy of your friends! And let's not forget that research has proved that your baby, too, will benefit in many ways from all your efforts.

On top of all the physical benefits, what I hope you will also take from this book is the mental strength that will see both you and your baby through this marvellous experience (morning sickness, intense fatigue, leaky boobs, mood swings, labour pain and all) and help aid your recovery after your baby is born.

I wish you the best of luck with your delivery – having taken on board the guidance in this book you may be confident that you have prepared well. Yes it hurts, but many of us do it time and time again, and I am sure that with a little bit of luck and the great care available to you from those angels and saints we call midwives, all will be well in the end. Your baby is going to come out one way or another ...

I would like to write more here about exercises that will help you during labour, and how to deal with that whole experience, but that's another book entirely! Indeed there is much more I would have liked to include in this book, but there are only so many pages, and there are many other books available, written by experts in this field, that can guide you through the final stages of your pregnancy and your post-natal recovery period.

I hope that what this book has done is to point you in the right direction with regard to what exercise to do, or not do, during your pregnancy. I am sure you are now armed with the knowledge and information you need to help you find a good instructor. There are many good pre- and post-natal exercise teachers out there: I know because I have met and trained quite a few of them, so go out and use them and, who knows, if you decide to have another baby you may well find yourself reading my next book!

Whatever lies ahead for you, embrace your wonderful, beautiful, clever body and give your new little one a kiss from me when you see them.

Appendix: Physical problems in pregnancy

This section provides information on some conditions that you may experience during pregnancy. It is not meant to be an exhaustive list, as that would constitute another book entirely; however these are all conditions that mean you may have to adapt or alter your current exercise programme.

Major physical problems

Symphysis pubis dysfunction

The pelvis is made up of the illium, ischium and pubis. The pelvic bones are joined at the back by the sacrum, forming the sacroiliac joints. The pelvic bones are joined at the front, forming the pubic symphysis. The two sides are joined at the front of the pelvis by discs of fibro-cartilage. This helps to form a cartilaginous joint that in a non-pregnant state does not actually move.

As we already know, pregnancy hormones relax the ligaments and therefore make joints less stable. The sacroiliac joint has strong ligaments and the pubic symphysis has smaller ligaments to help protect and support the joint. During pregnancy, these ligaments are affected and become more pliable, therefore allowing some movement. These processes are essential during childbirth to help enlarge the pelvic outlet and aid the passage of the baby through the pelvis. It is quite normal in pregnancy for there to be a gap in the pubic symphysis. Ultrasound scans have shown normal gaps of up to 4 mm, however gaps can increase to approximately 9 mm. The size and severity of the gap may cause pain down the front of the pelvis. For some, the pain may be considerable and they may find even simple movements such as walking difficult. Activities such as getting in and out of the bath may become practically impossible without help. Walking up a flight of stairs or getting into a car may cause great discomfort. If you are unlucky enough to have these symptoms, you may be suffering from symphysis pubis dysfunction. Most women find this condition a problem after pregnancy in particular, as damage can occur during labour. However, some mums-to-be also suffer from this condition and find that their quality of life and general mobility is greatly reduced.

'Clicking' in the joints may be a symptom, you may also adopt a waddling gait when walking. Some mums-to-be may even have to walk with a Zimmer frame or are advised to take bed rest to avoid weight-bearing on the pelvis. If you do feel that you have any problems with your pelvis beyond the normal aches and pains of pregnancy, then I would suggest that you see your GP and ask for referral to a physiotherapist who specialises in women's health. The right sort of physiotherapy-based exercise may help, but unfortunately general exercise may only exacerbate the condition.

During pregnancy it is not uncommon to experience some sort of discomfort around the pelvis, either at the front or back. However, you should not have any extreme pain or discomfort, specifically in the middle part of the pubic symphysis. Symptoms may be sudden and painful, or there may be constant tenderness and aching down the front of the pubic bone and down the inside of the thighs. While it is the front of the pelvis that can separate during pregnancy, this will also have a destabilising effect on the sacroiliac joint and you may get pain around the sacroiliac joint or lower back.

If you look at the section on running (see pages 80–81) you will note that you can run throughout your pregnancy (if you are already used to running, use good-quality training shoes and run on soft even ground). However, as the pelvis is unstable in pregnancy activities such as running or breaststroke swimming may exacerbate separation of the pelvis and cause greater pain in the sacroiliac area if you have symptoms of this condition. You are likely to see swimming recommended as an ideal form of exercise in pregnancy, but breaststroke should be avoided if you suffer from this condition.

It is important that during your pregnancy you avoid excessive stretching and any activity that calls for the legs to be taken out to a wide position. Exercises that are fast and involve quick changes of position should be avoided as they could encourage separation of the pelvis. Avoid overuse of one leg or unstable positions requiring balance.

Exercises that help to condition the deep abdominals (the core muscles) and that work the pelvic stability muscles are useful in preventing separation of the pelvis as they will help keep the stabilising muscles of the body strong to help support and protect the pelvis. (See Chapters 6 and 16, on core stability and Pilates, respectively.)

Low blood pressure

In some cases, the hormonal effects of pregnancy can lead to low blood pressure during the early stages. Care is therefore needed when changing positions or getting up from and down to the floor during your exercise sessions and, indeed, in everyday life. Your blood pressure should return to normal as you move into the second trimester.

High blood pressure

If you have high blood pressure you should not exercise and will be under constant medical supervision. High blood pressure in pregnancy can be life-threatening to both mum-to-be and baby. In some cases the vessels in the body don't stretch and may contract, causing the blood pressure to rise. This is known as pregnancy-induced hypertension.

Symptoms that occur with increased blood pressure can be blurred vision, sudden swelling and 'stars' before your eyes, severe headaches and, at times, a pain in the side. If you have any of these symptoms, avoid exercise and consult your healthcare provider. It is worth noting that during cardiovascular exercise your blood pressure will rise but only the systolic figure (the top figure) should be affected, this is normal and safe. This increase in the systolic blood pressure can remain after exercise but should subside and return to normal after about 15 minutes.

Supine hypotensive syndrome

This condition may affect you in the second and third trimesters, and while it can happen from 12 weeks of pregnancy, it is more likely to be a concern once the pregnancy is more advanced, at 16–20 weeks. As the pregnancy progresses the uterus enlarges, placing pressure on the inferior vena cava, specifically if you lay on your back to exercise. The vena cava is the vein responsible for returning blood to the heart from the body and legs. Lying on your back may restrict blood flow and can cause symptoms such as dizziness, nausea and claustrophobic feelings, breathing difficulties and, at worst, fainting. These symptoms are signs of supine hypotensive syndrome and should not be ignored as reducing the blood supply to the mother-to-be's brain may also mean there is a reduction of blood supply to the foetus. With any signs of supine hypotensive syndrome you should turn on to your left-hand side. Stop exercising on your back immediately and avoid doing so until after delivery.

You should be aware of supine hypotensive syndrome throughout your pregnancy. Not only can this condition affect you when you lie on your back, it may also affect you when you sit or stand still for some time. If you keep still, your circulation eventually slows down and blood may pool in your legs. This may restrict blood flow around your body and, consequently, restrict blood flow to the foetus. This may make you feel light-headed. It may even cause you to faint as a way of getting you to lie down so that blood circulation round the body can return to normal, thus restarting supply to the foetus. Not pleasant I know, but very clever!

To conclude, when you are exercising, make sure that you do not stand still for any length of time. For instance, when doing upper-body exercises sit rather than stand as you get heavier, or alternate an upper-body exercise where your legs are still with a lower-body exercise where you move your legs. If you are doing a yoga or Pilates class that involves many standing postures together, ensure that you move your legs whenever possible in order to maintain your circulation.

If you are one of those mums-to-be who can only get to sleep when lying on your back (and, let's face it, sleeping on your tummy is probably going to become impossible at some point) then please don't worry – you should be propped up with pillows and if you feel OK there is no need for alarm or cause for concern. Some of your antenatal checks may well be done with you on your back but, again, you will be propped up and kept in this position for the minimum amount of time.

Diastasis
See pages 28–9.

Breast discomfort
Some exercise positions may need to be adapted if you have any breast tenderness, as well as to accommodate the growing size of the breast. This can be a problem at any stage of pregnancy, but specifically in the early and late stages.

You may need to wear breast pads towards the end of pregnancy, particularly when exercising. When performing any type of aerobic activity (apart from swimming), a good and supportive sports bra should be worn. Always avoid exercising without supporting the breasts, or exercising in an underwired bra while pregnant – as your breasts will be heavier than usual, there is more chance of stretching your Cooper's ligaments, which are the ones that help support the breasts.

Carpal tunnel syndrome

Carpal tunnel syndrome is something that can affect some women in pregnancy. This is a result of the effect of pregnancy hormones on the body; these bring about changes in the blood volume that can cause swelling of the wrist, thus applying pressure on the nerves. This can lead to tingling, numbness or stiffness in the hands. Carpal tunnel syndrome can affect women pre- and post-natally at any time. It is, however, more likely to occur at around 24 weeks, as you will tend to retain more fluid at this time. It may cause pain or tingling in the wrists and hands. You may find that it becomes difficult to open jars or pick up small objects, say. Women often say that their symptoms are at their worst in the morning or later in the evening. If you suffer from carpal tunnel syndrome you need to avoid exercising in positions where the weight is borne on the hands; gripping tightly may also aggravate the condition. Do take extra care, too, when picking up hot drinks or pans.

You may find that using small dumbbells instead of tubing or resistance bands is less stressful on the wrist. Using weight-training gloves during rowing activities or indoor cycling classes may also help.

It is important at any time to use the correct wrist and hand positions when exercising, but never more so than during pregnancy. Incorrect positioning of the wrist when weight training, for instance, will place inappropriate pressure on the wrists.

If you are suffering symptoms of carpal tunnel syndrome you must seek advice from your health professional. Putting your hands in iced water and moving the fingers, though not very pleasant may help reduce some of the symptoms. If it helps, I suggest you do this and then place your freezing hands on your partner at regular intervals, as this will also help to take your mind off the pain!

Braxton Hicks contractions

These are practice contractions when there is a tightening of the abdominal area with mild period-type pains in the lower abdomen. They can occur any time and while they are a normal and necessary symptom of pregnancy, it is best to avoid exercising while experiencing them.

Occasionally, some mums-to-be find that exercising brings on Braxton Hicks contractions, and while there is no research to explain this, the condition should be monitored and your exercise programme adapted as necessary.

Diabetes

Diabetes can greatly affect the health and well-being of your baby. If you are diabetic before pregnancy or you get gestational diabetes during pregnancy, you will need to get your blood glucose levels checked regularly. Exercise is a demand that is superimposed on the existing condition, and any exercise programme needs to be managed and guided by your healthcare provider or GP. However, it is well documented that regular exercise can help in controlling diabetes, by increasing your maximum oxygen uptake and decreasing your blood pressure. Both these effects can help in controlling blood glucose levels.

Weight gain

Weight gain is a normal and necessary part of being pregnant. During my pregnancies I put on the recommended two stone each time, give or take a few pounds, and I looked huge! This was just the way I carried my babies. I exercised all the way through my pregnancies, had great deliveries and could breast-feed for Great Britain. It is important, though, that you don't put on excessive weight during pregnancy; and we must accept that everybody is different. We will all gain weight differently, we will all carry our babies differently, and we will all look different. Looking pregnant is beautiful! Some authorities say that you should put on three to four pounds during the first two months of pregnancy. However, this is a very individual matter. Many of you may not gain any weight at all; some of you may even lose weight if you have bad sickness. Others may put on more weight in the early stages. Everybody is different. The bigger picture we need to look at is the overall weight you gain during pregnancy.

The American National Academy of Sciences advises that you gain between 25 and 35 pounds during pregnancy if you were a normal weight before conceiving. If you were overweight before pregnancy, then 15–25 pounds may be a more appropriate weight gain. While those who are obese may look at gaining 15 pounds throughout their pregnancy, underweight mums-to-be may gain between 28 and 40 pounds. Remember: these are guidelines only.

I hope this book helps you to look after yourself, stay fit and well and avoid too much weight gain, but remember that weight gain is a normal and necessary factor of pregnancy. Remember at all times that the weight you gain is not permanent.

Research has concluded that women who exercise throughout their pregnancy gain less weight and less body fat than other mums who do no exercise other than normal daily activities. The exercising group did, however, gain a normal healthy amount of weight.

Women who are underweight at the time they get pregnant and then gain too little weight during pregnancy may be more likely to deliver babies a little early and have babies with reduced birth weight (less than 5.5 pounds). Babies born early and babies that have low birth weight are more prone to health problems.

All this said, don't reach for the biscuit tin! Excessive weight gain can be dangerous. Those who are overweight before pregnancy and/or gain excessive weight are more likely to develop high blood pressure, pre-eclampsia or gestational diabetes.

pregnant. Yet by the end of the first trimester Sarah had developed some very large and quite painful varicose veins. This was just the way her body reacted to the changes. The good thing is that they did reduce once she had her baby.

Varicose veins do not only occur in the legs: you may develop them in the vulva too. Haemorrhoids (piles) are just varicose veins that occur in the rectum. Should you suffer from these, you should avoid exercises that put pressure on the area, such as cycling, or at least use a well-padded seat.

Here are a few important points to bear in mind.

- Regular exercise helps increase the circulation and maintain muscle tone.
- Avoid standing or sitting for long periods of time.
- Avoid crossing your legs.
- Avoid excessive weight gain.
- Use support tights if necessary, but not when exercising.

Low back pain

This book contains lots of information about your posture and the physical adaptations that your baby makes during pregnancy. With all this in mind, is it any wonder that we get back pain in pregnancy? The joints become unstable and the centre of gravity changes. The muscles of the abdominals become stretched and can 'gap' (diastasis recti); this all means that the back has limited support. To help prevent or alleviate back pain, read the sections in this book on posture and diastasis (see pages 34 and 28–9).

If you need some immediate relief, try resting by lying down rather than sitting. Place a pillow between your legs or under your tummy to help you get as comfortable as you can. Massage may help, as may a hot water bottle in a pillowcase placed against your lower back. Use of a maternity belt when doing housework and so on can be useful but should not be an excuse for forgetting your core stability exercises.

Getting on all-fours to do the following exercise can help alleviate back pain, both during your pregnancy and in labour. You can use a stability ball or chair at home. Kneel on a pillow or folded towel, resting your head and arms on either the chair or ball. Slightly contract your abdominals, tilt your pelvis under then release it a few times. Try rocking your body from side to side and forwards and backwards (it is better to use a ball for this as it will fit around you and move more easily when rocking).

If the pain is severe then do consult your GP, who may refer you to an obstetric physiotherapist.

Tension in the neck and upper shoulders

The increasing size of your breasts can affect the way you hold yourself. As your tummy grows your centre of gravity changes, and without work on your posture you may find that you round your upper back to help maintain your balance. This results in the neck shifting forwards. The muscles at the back of the neck then become shorter and tighter, while the muscles at the front of the neck become longer and weaker. Tightness in the neck extensor muscles causes tension around the neck and shoulders. It can also decrease circulation – not to any dangerous degree, but it may cause headaches, tension and the like.

Join a good beginners' Pilates class or a specific pregnancy and exercise class. Both should work on training to maintain good posture. This will involve exercises to strengthen the muscles between the shoulder blades and the muscles that help to stabilise your shoulder blades; stretching the chest muscles may also help. Always wear a good and supportive bra, remind yourself to relax your shoulders and keep a good upper-body posture as much as possible. Exercise in general can help relieve tension and loosen tight shoulders, as well as producing 'feel-good' hormones. A massage of the neck and shoulders, or a warm wheat bag placed across the neck and shoulders may also help.

Fatigue

Tiredness and fatigue are common symptoms of pregnancy. You will often feel tired in the early and very late stages of pregnancy. For every hour you spend exercising you should spend at least half that time resting. During my first pregnancy I taught classes in the morning and in the evening so that, in the afternoon, I could come home and watch a regular 20-minute soap. I would switch off the phone and close the curtains. Once my baby was born, she would become very quiet and relaxed whenever she heard the theme tune!

Rest is an important aspect of caring for yourself and your baby during pregnancy. Your body is very busy growing and providing for your unborn baby, and is one of the most important and physically demanding jobs you will ever have.

Bibliography

Total Core Strength on the Ball
Cherry Baker
MQ Publications, 2004

The Complete Guide to Postnatal Fitness
(2nd edition)
Judy DiFore
A & C Black, 2003

Exercising Through Your Pregnancy
James F. Clapp III MD
Addicus Books, 2002

Abdominal Training (2nd edition)
Christopher M. Norris
A & C Black, 2001

The Food Guide Pyramid
Champaign, Human Nutrition Information Services
USA Department of Agriculture, 1992

Back Stability
Christopher M. Norris
Human Kinetics, 2000

Fit for Two
Thomas W. Hanlon
Human Kinetics, 1995

Maternal Fitness
Julie Tupler
Prentice Hall, 1996

Bodytoning
Christopher M. Norris
A & C Black, 2003

Expecting Fitness
Birgitta Gallo
Renaissance Books, 2000

Fit to Deliver
Karen Nordahl, Susi Kerr and Carl Pertersen
Fit to Deliver Intl, 2000

What to Expect When You're Expecting
(3rd edition)
Arlene Eisenberg
Simon & Schuster, 2002

The Prenatal Exercise Handbook
Jenny Whitby
Sidgwick & Jackson Ltd, 1989

Useful addresses and websites

Modern Pilates
9a Cleasby Rd
Menston
Nr Ilkley
West Yorkshire LS29 6JE
www.modernpilates.co.uk

Pregnancy Personal Training and Teacher Training
The Studio
Surrey Street
Glossop
Derbyshire SK13 7AY
www.thestudioglossop.co.uk

Guild of Pregnancy and Postnatal Exercise Instructors
www.postnatalexercise.co.uk

YMCA Fitness Industry Training
111 Great Russell Street
London WC1B 3NP
www.ymcafit.org

Pregnant Pilates Training For Midwifes and Health Professionals
Modern Pilates
9a Cleasby Rd
Menston
Nr Ilkley
West Yorkshire LS29 6JE
www.modernpilates.co.uk

The Register of Exercise Professionals
8–10 Crown Hill
Croydon
Surrey CR0 1RZ
www.exerciseregister.org

Aqua Fusion
Northern Fitness and Education
9a Cleasby Rd
Menston
Nr Ilkley
West Yorkshire LS29 6JE
www.aquafusion.co.uk

The National Childbirth Trust
Alexandra House
Oldham Terrace
Acton
London W3 6NH
www.nctpregnancyandbabycare.com

The Continence Foundation
307 Hatton Square
16 Baldwins Gardens
London EC1N 7RJ
www.continence-foundation.org.uk

British Symphysis Pubis Dysfunction Support Group
c/o National Childbirth Trust (see above)
www.spd-uk.org

The Association of Chartered Physiotherapists in Women's Health
www.acpwh.org.uk

The Miscarriage Association
c/o Clayton Hospital
Northgate
Wakefield
West Yorkshire WF1 3JS
www.miscarriageassociation.org.uk

The Active Birth Centre
25 Bickerton Road
London N19 5JT
www.activebirthcentre.com

Stillbirth and Neonatal Death Society
28 Portland Place
London W1B 1LY
www.uk-sands.org

Index